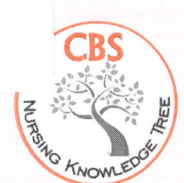

Integrated Supervised

INTERNSHIP

for GNM Third Year Part-II

(As per the New Syllabus of INC for GNM Students)

Taranpreet Kaur

BSc Medical, MBA (Marketing) , MSc Nursing (Community Health Nursing)

Associate Professor
College of Nursing (Adesh Institute of Medical Sciences and Research)
Sri Muktsar Sahib, Punjab, India

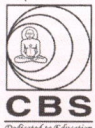

CBS
Dedicated to Education

CBS Publishers & Distributors Pvt Ltd

• New Delhi • Bengaluru • Chennai • Kochi • Mumbai
• Hyderabad • Kolkata • Nagpur • Patna • Vijayawada

Integrated Supervised

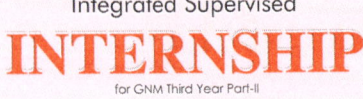

INTERNSHIP

for GNM Third Year Part-II

ISBN: 978-93-88108-89-8

Reprint: 2021

First Edition: 2019

Published by **Satish Kumar Jain** and produced by **Varun Jain** for

CBS Publishers & Distributors Pvt Ltd

4819/XI Prahlad Street, 24 Ansari Road, Daryaganj, New Delhi 110 002, India.
Ph: +91-11-23289259, 23266861, 23266867   Website: www.cbspd.com
Fax: 011-23243014
e-mail: delhi@cbspd.com; cbspubs@airtelmail.in.

Corporate Office: 204 FIE, Industrial Area, Patparganj, Delhi 110 092
Ph: +91-11-4934 4934   Fax: 4934 4935
e-mail: feedback@cbspd.com; bhupesharora@cbspd.com

Branches

- **Bengaluru:** Seema House 2975, 17th Cross, K.R. Road, Banasankari 2nd Stage, Bengaluru 560 070, Karnataka
  Ph: +91-80-26771678/79   Fax: +91-80-26771680   e-mail: bangalore@cbspd.com
- **Chennai:** 7, Subbaraya Street, Shenoy Nagar, Chennai 600 030, Tamil Nadu
  Ph: +91-44-26680620, 26681266   Fax: +91-44-42032115   e-mail: chennai@cbspd.com
- **Kochi:** 68/1534, 35, 36-Power House Road, Opp. KSEB, Cochin-682018, Kochi, Kerala
  Ph: +91-484-4059061-65   Fax: +91-484-4059065   e-mail: kochi@cbspd.com
- **Kolkata:** 6/B, Ground Floor, Rameswar Shaw Road, Kolkata-700 014, West Bengal
  Ph: +91-33-22891126, 22891127, 22891128   e-mail: kolkata@cbspd.com
- **Mumbai:** PWD Shed, Gala No. 25/26, Ramchandra Bhatt Marg, Next to J.J. Hospital Gate No. 2,
  Opp. Union Bank of India, Noor Baug, Mumbai-400009
  Ph: +91-22-66661880/89   Fax: +91-22-24902342   e-mail: mumbai@cbspd.com

Representatives

- **Hyderabad**   +91-9885175004
- **Pune**   +91-9623451994
- **Patna**   +91-9334159340
- **Vijayawada**   +91-9000660880

Printed at: Goyal Offset Works Pvt. Ltd.

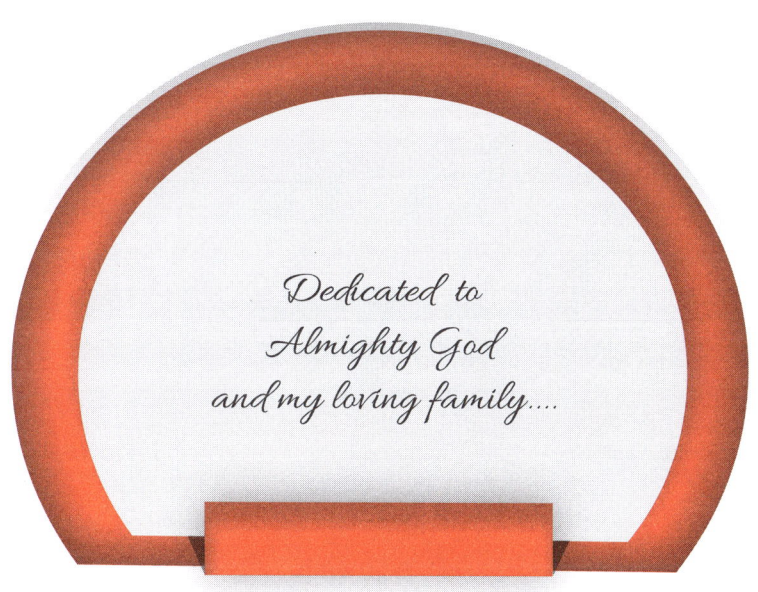

Dedicated to
Almighty God
and my loving family....

Reviewers' List

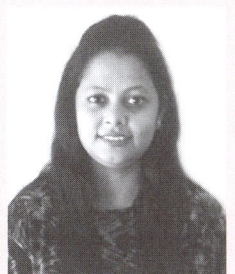

Priyanka Randhir BSc(N) RN RM

Nursing Tutor
SMLD School of Nursing
Amritsar, Punjab
India

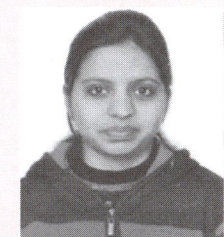

Miss Timsy MSc Nursing (Obstetrics and Gynecology)

Assistant Professor
Desh Bhagat University, Mandi Gobindgarh, Punjab, India

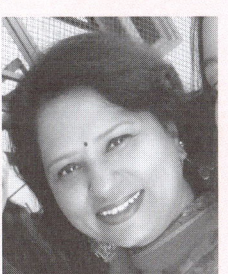

Anju Dhir BSc Science MSc Microbiology, PhD Biotechnology,

Lecturer (Microbiology)
Shivalik Institute of Nursing Shimla, Himachal Pradesh, India

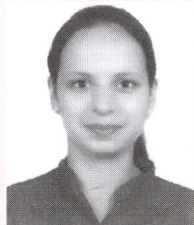

Eenu MS Nursing (Community Health Nursing)

Maharishi Markandeshwar Deemed to be University Mullana, Ambala, Haryana

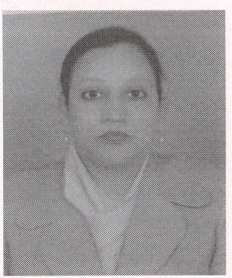

Devinder Kaur MSc (Medical Surgical Nursing)

Principal
Gian Sagar College of Nursing, Punjab, India

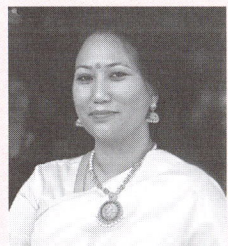

Suman Bodh MSc (Community Health Nursing)

Principal
GNM Training School
Dr RPGMC Tanda

Preface

The idea of presenting this book to nursing world is to put the existing knowledge and modern concept of nursing in India. This book contains contents useful for nursing students. It is an attempt to cover modern thoughts with the latest curriculum prepared by the Indian Nursing Council for the internship of general nursing and midwifery.

This book is divided into four sections:

- Nursing Education
- Introduction to Research and Statistics
- Professional Trends and Adjustment
- Nursing Administration and Ward Management.

Each part fulfills the general objectives of the subject. Being nursing teacher it is quite easy for me to understand the difficulties of students. I have made a humble effort to meet those difficulties as far as possible. I hope this book will benefit immensely to all diploma and undergraduate students. Although, I have done my level best but there may be some discrepancies, your valuable suggestions are always welcome.

Taranpreet Kaur

Acknowledgements

"You'll meet more angels on a winding path than on a straight one"

—*Terri Guillemets*

The successful completion of this manuscript was possible through the invaluable contribution of a number of people. Saying thank you is not enough to express my gratitude.

The first offering of gratitude goes to Almighty God for keeping me on track, motivating me, when I felt exhausted, never leaving me alone in my emptiness.

My deep gratitude to my husband Er. Manwinder Singh, my family and those loved ones who inspired me and keep motivating me.

A very special thanks to my ever loving friend and Bhabi Ms Davinder Kaur for her guidance and motivation for writing and completing this book from time to time.

I wish to express my appreciation and gratitude to all my colleagues who spared their valuable time and helped me throughout.

My special thanks to my daughter Arashgeet Kaur and my son Manavgeet Singh for giving me time and positive energy to complete this book.

I would also like to thank Mr Satish Kumar Jain (Chairman) and Mr Varun Jain (Managing Director), M/s CBS Publishers and Distributors Pvt Ltd for providing me the platform in bringing out the book. I have no words to describe the role, efforts, inputs and initiatives undertaken by Mr Bhupesh Arora Vice President-Publishing and Marketing, PGMEE and Nursing Division for helping and motivating me.

I thank Mr Anubhav Puri (Assistant Territory Sales Manages) who persuaded me to write this book, which is one more step in my writing carrier

I especially thank Dr Mrinalini Bakshi (Senior Content Developer and Editor) for her editorial support and Ms Nitasha Arora (Project Manager), Ms Neetu Jindal (Asst. Production Manager), Mr Nitish K Dubey (Senior Editor) and all the production team members Ms Tahira Praveen, Mr Ashutosh Pathak, Mr Prakash Gaur, Mr Chaman Lal, Mr Phool Kumar, Mr Bunty Kashyap, Ms Babita Verma, Mr Raju Sharma, Mr Manoj Chaudhary, Mr Vikram Chaudhary and Manoj Malakar for devoting laborious hours in designing and typesetting of this book.

Syllabus for
GNM Students

NURSING EDUCATION, INTRODUCTION TO RESEARCH, PROFESSIONAL TRENDS & ADJUSTMENT & NURSING ADMINISTRATION & WARD MANAGEMENT

Placement: Internship (3rd Years Part II)   Time: 120 Hours

NURSING EDUCATION

Course Description

This course is designed to introduce the students to the concept of teaching as an integral part of nursing practice.

Total Hours: 20

Unit	Learning objectives	Contents	Hrs	Teaching learning activities	Method of Assessment
I	Describe the concept of education	**Introduction** • Education ▪ Meaning, aims, scopeand purposes,	2	Lecture cum discussion	Short answers Objective type
II	Explain the process of teaching and learning	**Teaching learning process** • Basic principles • Characteristics of teaching and learning • Teaching responsibility of a nurse • Preparation of teaching plan	4	Lecture cum discussion	Short answers Objective type Evaluation of teaching plan
III	Narrate the methods of teaching Describe the clinical teaching methods	**Methods of teaching** • Methods of teaching • Clinical teaching methods ▪ Case method ▪ Bed side clinic ▪ Nursing rounds ▪ Nursing conference (individual and group) ▪ Process recording.	14	Lecture cum discussion	Short answer Objective type Evaluation of planned as well as incidental health teaching

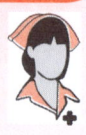

INTRODUCTION TO RESEARCH

Course Description:

This course is designed to develop fundamental abilities and attitude in the students towards scientific methods of investigation and utilization of research finding so as to improve practice of nursing.

Total Hours: 30

Unit	Learning Objectives	Contents	Hrs	Teaching learning activities	Assessment Method
I	Discuss the importance of research in Nursing	**Introduction** • Definition • Terminology related to research • Need and importance of nursing research • Characteristics of good research	3	Lecture cum discussion	Short answers Objective type
II	Describe the research process	**Research process** • Purposes and objectives • Steps in research process	3	Lecture cum discussion	Short answer Essay type
III	Describe the various research approaches	**Research approaches and designs** • Types • Methods • Advantages and disadvantages	5	Lecture cum discussion	Short answer Essay type
IV	Describe the various data collection methods	**Data collection process** • Meaning • Methods and instruments of data collection	5	Lecture cum discussion	Short answer Essay type
V	List the steps involved in data analysis	**Analysis of data** • Compilation • Tabulation • Classification • Summarization • Presentation and interpretation of data using descriptive statistic	6	Lecture cum discussion Reading the research articles	Short answer Essay type

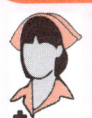

Unit	Learning Objectives	Contents	Hrs	Teaching learning activities	Assessment Method
VI	Describe the importance of statistics in research	**Introduction to statistics** • Definition • Use of statistics • Scales of measurement • Frequency distribution • Mean, median, mode and standard deviation.	6	Lecture cum discussion	Short answer Essay type
VII	Describe the utilization of research in nursing practice	**Utilization of research in nursing practice** • Evidence based practice	2	Lecture cum discussion	Short answer Essay type

PROFESSIONAL TRENDS AND ADJUSTMENT

Course Description

This course is designed to help students develop an understanding of the career opportunities available for professional development.

S. No	Learning objectives	Contents	Hrs	Teaching learning activities	Assessment methods
I	Describe nursing as a profession	**Nursing as a profession** • Definition of profession • Criteria of a profession and nursing profession • Evolution of Nursing Profession in India • Educational preparation of a professional nurse • Qualities/ Characteristics and role of a professional nurse	4	Lecture cum discussion	Short answer Objective type Essay type
II	Explain various aspects of Professional ethics	**Professional ethics** • Meaning and relationship of professional ethics and etiquettes • Code of ethics for nurse by ICN • Standards for nursing practice (INC) • Etiquettes for employment: locating posting, applying and accepting a position, resignation from a position.	6	Lecture cum discussion Assignment: Application for job acceptance & job resignation	Short answer Essay type

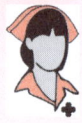

S. No	Learning objectives	Contents	Hrs	Teaching learning activities	Assessment methods
III	Discuss the importance of continuing education in personal and professional development	**Personal and professional development** • Continuing education ▪ Meaning and importance ▪ Scope ▪ Identifying opportunities	10	Lecture cum discussion	Short answer Essay type
		• Career in Nursing ▪ Opportunities available in Nursing in Hospital, Community teaching and other related special organization. • In-service education ▪ Definition ▪ Value ▪ Need participation in committee procedures ▪ Nursing in the future		Draw a career ladder in nursing in reference to international influence and financial aid.	
IV	Discuss the significance of legislation in Nursing	**Legislation in nursing** • Purpose and importance of laws in Nursing • Legal Terms • Common legal hazards in Nursing • Laws and regulations related to health care providers in India at different levels • Service and institutional rules • Regulation of nursing education • Registration and reciprocities	5	Lecture cum discussion	Assignment

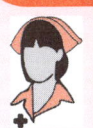

S. No	Learning objectives	Contents	Hrs	Teaching learning activities	Assessment methods

V	List the various organizations related to health and nursing profession and briefly describe their function	**Profession and related organizations**
		• Regulatory bodies: Indian Nursing Council, State Nursing Council
		• Professional organizations:
		  ▪ Trained Nurses Association of India,
		  ▪ Students Nurses Association,
		  ▪ Nurses League of the Christian Medical Association of India,
		  ▪ International Council of Nurses (ICN),
		  ▪ International Confederation of Midwives etc.
		• Related organization and their contribution to nursing: World Health Organization, Red cross and St. john's Ambulance, Colombo plan, UNICEF, World Bank etc.
			5	Lecture cum discussion
				
				Observational visits to State Nursing Council and Local TNAI office
					Report of visit to the council
					
					Short answers Essay type

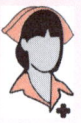

NURSING ADMINISTRATION AND WARD MANAGEMENT

Course Description

This course is designed to help the student to understand the basic principles of administration and its application to the management of ward and health care unit.

Unit	Learning Objectives	Contents	Hrs	Teaching learning activities	Assessment methods
I	Describe the meaning, philosophy and principles of administration	**Introduction** • Administration and management ▪ Meaning ▪ Philosophy ▪ Elements and principles ▪ Significance	4	Lecture cum discussion	Short answers Objective type Essay type
II	Describe the management process	**Management process** • Planning ▪ Importance ▪ Purpose ▪ Types of planning • Organization ▪ Principles of organization ▪ Organization chart of hospital/ ward/ PHC/ Sub center • Staffing ▪ Scheduling ▪ Recruitment, selection, deployment, retaining, promotion, superannuation ▪ Personnel management ▪ Job description ▪ Job specification ▪ Staff development and staff welfare • Directing • Co-ordination and control ▪ Quality management • Budgeting • Policies of hospital and various department of the hospital	15	Lecture cum discussion Companion of organization charts	Short answers Essay type Objective type Written test Evaluation of the organization chart prepared by students.

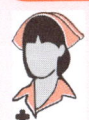

Unit	Learning Objectives	Contents	Hrs	Teaching learning activities	Assessment methods
IV	Explain the administration of different health care units	**Administration of hospital/ department/unit/ ward** • Health centre/ unit physical layout • Safety measures for prevention of accidents and infections • Legal responsibilities of a nurse • Leadership styles • Problem solving : process and approach, steps and methods of dealing with complaints of patients and other health team members. • Records and reports: meaning, types, importance.	9	Lecture cum discussion Role play Group work on physical layout Reading notes	Short answers Objective type Essay type
V	Discuss the importance of maintaining supplies and equipment for effective administration	**Management of equipment supplies.** • Maintenance of supplies & equipment (preventive maintenance) • Handing over and taking over of inventory • Indent and ordering of supplies and equipment • Problem solving : process and approach, steps and methods of dealing with supplies and equipment.	7	Lecture cum discussion Role play Group project on problem solving	Short answers Objective type Essay type Evaluation of the report on Group project
VI	Discuss the cost and financing of health services in India	**Cost and financing of health care** • Cost of health care • Health financing • National health plans (annual and five year plans) and outlays, role of state and central government in allocation of funds • Health insurance- types, issues etc.	5	Lecture cum discussion	Short answer Test

Contents

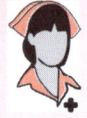

SECTION 4: NURSING ADMINISTRATION AND WARD MANAGEMENT

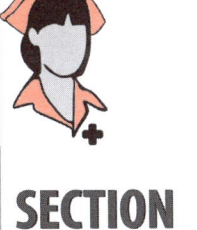

SECTION 1

NURSING EDUCATION

- ➲ Introduction to Education

- ➲ Teaching-Learning Process

- ➲ Methods of Teaching

Introduction to Education

1

Learning Objectives

- To describe the concept of education.
- To explain about the nursing education.

Key Terms

- **Education:** The process of receiving or giving systematic instructions, especially at a school or university.
- **Knowledge:** Facts, Information and skills acquired through experience or education.

INTRODUCTION

Education word is derived from two Latin words *Educare* and *Educere*, where *Educare* means 'to nourish, to bring up, to rise' and *Educere* means 'to bring forth, to lead out or to draw out'. In broader sense education means 'the act of teaching and training'.

DEFINITIONS

- The manifestation of divine perfection existing in man. Education means the exposition of man's complete individuality.
  —*Swami Vivekananda*
- Education is the realization of the self.
  —*Shankaracharya*
- By education, I mean all round drawing out the best in the child and man-body, mind and spirit.
  —*Gandhiji*
- Enabling the mind to find out that ultimate truth which emancipates us from the bondage of dust and gives us the wealth, not of things but of inner light, not of power but of love, making truth its own and giving expression to it.
  —*Tagore*
- Education as a means of character formation and righteous living.
  —*Swami Dayanand*

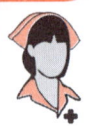

- Education means self-realization and service of people.
  —Guru Nanak Devji
- Education means training for country and love for nation. *—Chanakya*
- Education is the development of the power of adaptation to ever changing social environment. *—PC Bannerji*
- Education is the capacity to feel pleasure and pain, at the right moment. It developed the body and the soul of the pupil, all the beauty and all the perfection which he is capable of. *—Plato*
- Education is something which makes a man self-reliant and selfless.
  —Rigveda

AIMS AND PURPOSES OF EDUCATION

Aims are one which gives direction to the education which is a planned and purposeful activity.

Factors Determining Aims of Education

- Philosophy of life
- Elements of human
- Religious factors
- Political ideologies
- Socioeconomic factors and problems of country
- Cultural factors
- Exploration of knowledge

General aims of education are as follows (Fig. 1):

- **Vocational efficiency** through education helps to earn livelihood and self-sufficiency. It gives economic and social independence.
- **Knowledge** is essential for intellectual growth, good interpersonal relationship (IPR) and healthy adjustment in life. These can be attained by the knowledge and education.
- **Complete living:** Self-preservation, performance of social, political, beneficial, economic responsibilities of the part of human life. Education acquaints the person with activities of complete living.
- **Harmonious personality development:** Physical, intellectual emotional, mental, moral characters are well-balanced with education.
- **Self-realization:** Education should help a person, based on his potentialities, what a person is going to become.
- **Cultural development:** A person becomes civilized and cultured with education.
- **Citizenship:** A baby starts taking education to become a civilized citizen of the country.
- **Leisure:** Leisure is a complete part of human being. Education gives the direction to utilize the leisure time in creative and useful manner.

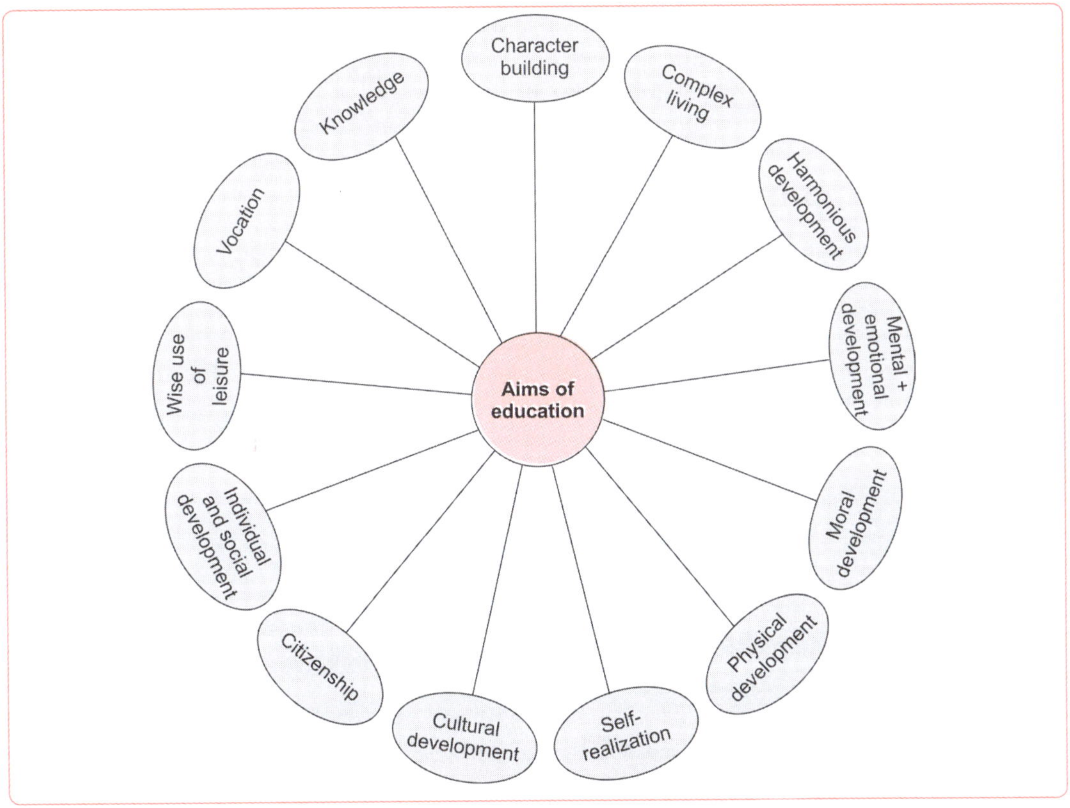

Fig. 1: Aims of education

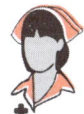

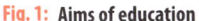

- **Development of leadership:** Education should train the youth to assume the leadership responsibilities. Initiating the students to the art of living is one of the educational aims.
- **Increased productivity:** Education helps the mankind by increasing the productivity with advanced scientific knowledge, technical ability and efficiency.
- **Social and national integration** with oneness and belongingness is educational aim.
- **Education helps in modernization** in all respects. People able to think, judge and implement their decisions efficiently.
- Education is for equality.

The National Education Policy of 1986 have set the following educational aims of our country which are still in force. They are:

- All round material and spiritual development of all people.
- Cultural orientation and development of interest in Indian culture.
- Scientific temper.
- National cohesion.
- Independence of mind and spirit.

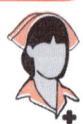

- ❏ Furthering the goals of socialism, secularism and democracy.
- ❏ Manpower development for different levels of economy.
- ❏ Fostering research in all areas of development.
- ❏ Education for equality.

SCOPE OF EDUCATION

Scope means the breadth, comprehensiveness, variety of learning experiences to be provided in the educational process. It refers to the extent of the range of view outlook. In fact, the scope of the education is very wide. It is the theme of life. It is dynamic force in the life of every individual, influencing his physical, mental, emotional, social and ethical development. We can say that scope is as wide as world and as long as the history of man on earth. On the whole education is must for understanding life and includes manners, values, morals, tasks and so on.

 ASSESS YOURSELF

1. Give different views of education.
2. Enlist the factors determining educational aims.
3. Write in detail the scope of education.

Teaching-Learning Process

2

Learning Objectives

- To explain the process of teaching and learning.
- To know the preparation of teaching plan.

Key Terms

- **Teacher:** Person who imparts knowledge to someone.
- **Student:** A learner.
- **Learning process:** The process of guiding the learner.
- **Responsibility:** Accountability.

INTRODUCTION

Teaching and learning are interdependent activities. They have four aspects as follows:

1. Teacher
2. Student
3. Learning process
4. Leaning situation

Teacher creates an aura for the learning of the students. They have the situation setup and interaction between them. Many variables like teacher, student, curriculum, laboratories and the studying environment are arranged in a systematic way to create a teaching-learning process.

CHIEF ASPECTS OF TEACHING-LEARNING PROCESS

- Command, planning and organization of subject matter or content and activities
- Class control and discipline
- Psychology of learners
- Evaluation

In fact, teaching and learning has a three way communication: Interaction between the teacher and learner is the core of teaching and learning process (Flow chart 1).

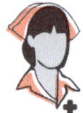

Flow chart 1: Teaching-learning process

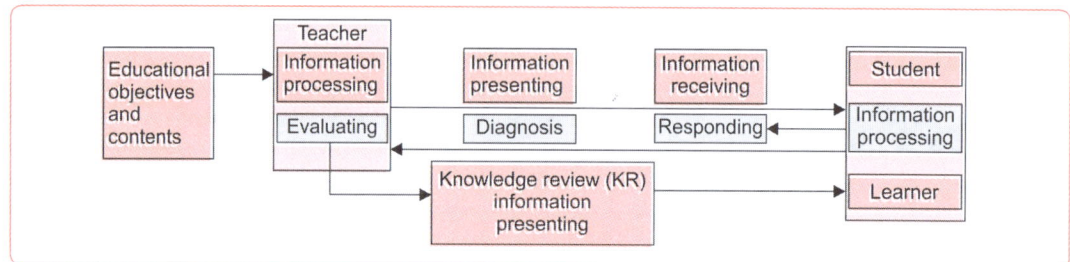

The process of guiding the learner involves eight steps as given in Flow chart 1. They are:

Step I — Educational objectives and content.

Step II — Communication from teacher to learner.

Step III — Receiving information from teacher to learner.

Step IV — Processing information in the learner.

Step V — Response from learner to teacher.

Step VI — Diagnosing learner by teacher.

Step VII — Formative evaluation of the learner by teacher.

Step VIII — Feedback information from teacher to learner.

BASIC PRINCIPLES OF LEARNING

❏ **Readiness:** Individuals learn best when they are ready to learn and they do not learn well if they see no reason for learning. Readiness implies a degree of single mindedness and eagerness, when students are ready to learn. They meet the instructor at least halfway, and this simplifies the instructor's job.

❏ **Exercise:** The principle of exercise states that those things most often repeated are the best remembers. It is the basis of drill and practice. The human memory in fallible, so practice makes a man perfect.

❏ **Effect:** The principle of effect is based on the emotional reaction of the student. It states that learning is strengthened when accompanied by a pleasant or satisfying feeling, and that learning is weakened when associated with an unpleasant feeling. Experiences that produce feeling of defeat, frustration, anger, confusion or futility are unpleasant for the student.

❏ **Primacy:** Primacy, the state of being first, often creates a strong, almost unshakable, impression for the instructor, this means that what is taught must be right the first time.

❏ **Intensity:** A vivid, dramatic, or exciting learning experience teachers more than a routine or boring experience. The principle of intensity implies that a student will learn more from the real thing than from a substitute.

❏ **Recency:** The principle of recency states that things most recently learned are best remembered. Conversely, the further a student is removed time wise from a new fact or understanding, the more difficult it is to remember. Instructors recognize the principle of recency when they carefully plan a summary for a ground school lesson. The principle of recency often determines the sequences of lectures within a course of instruction.

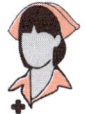

CHARACTERISTICS OF LEARNING

- ❏ Learning is unitary
- ❏ Learning is individual and social
- ❏ Learning is self-active
- ❏ Learning is purposive
- ❏ Learning is creative
- ❏ Learning is transferable
- ❏ Learning is organizing experience
- ❏ Learning is growth.

BASIC PRINCIPLES OF TEACHING

The educators and philosophers have emphasized certain principles of teaching which the teachers are expected to have in mind for making their teaching effective, efficient and inspirational.

- ❏ Principle of activity or learning by doing
- ❏ Principle of play way
- ❏ Principle of motivation
- ❏ Principle of self-education
- ❏ Principle of individual differences
- ❏ Principle of goal setting
- ❏ Principle of stimulation
- ❏ Principle of association
- ❏ Principle of readiness
- ❏ Principle of effect
- ❏ Principle of exercise or repetition
- ❏ Principle of changer and rest
- ❏ Principle of feedback and reinforcement
- ❏ Principle of training of senses
- ❏ Principle of group dynamics
- ❏ Principle of creativity
- ❏ Principle of correlation.

MAXIMS OF TEACHING

The term maxim of teaching may be defined as rules for presenting terms and concepts to make them easy to comprehensive in classroom teaching. They are the guidelines for teaching.

- ❏ Proceed from the known to unknown
- ❏ Proceed from simple to complex
- ❏ From easy to difficult
- ❏ Concrete to abstract

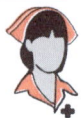

- From particular to general
- Analysis to synthesis
- From whole to parts
- From empirical to rational
- From psychological to logical
- Actual to the representative
- Indefinite to definite
- Near to far
- Inductivity.

NATURE AND CHARACTERISTICS OF TEACHING

- Teaching is a tri-polar process
- Teaching is an interactive process
- Teaching is both conscious and unconscious process
- Teaching is dynamic and is related to time and place
- Teaching guides the young and immature
- Teaching is a profession where teacher instructs and educate
- Teaching is an art and science
- Teaching is informal and formal which occurs outside and inside the class
- Teaching takes place in social setup
- Teaching is task oriented
- Teaching is observable through teacher-behavior or public teacher action
- Teaching is a therapy to learners
- Teaching is measurable and quantifiable by observational techniques
- Teaching is continuing from training to indoctrination
- Teaching stimulates the learners
- Teaching is training the emotions of the learner
- Teaching is dominated by communication skills
- Teaching is narrating, showing and doing
- Teaching is face to face encounter
- Teaching facilitates learning
- Teaching is modifiable by the use of mechanism of feedback devices
- Teaching is helping the learner to respond to his/her environment
- Teaching can be analyzed by following types: Pupil activity, learning components, learning conditions or structure, educational objectives, teacher activity.

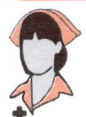

PREPARATION OF TEACHING PLAN

Lesson Plan

Planning is essential not only in teaching but in spheres of human activities. Lesson planning is an important part of planning of daily teaching. These are the brief outlines of the main point of the lesson. A teacher has to prepare more detailed, written plan.

Definitions

Lesson plan in the title given to a statement of the achievements to be realized and the specific meaning by which these are to be attained as a result of the activities engaged during the period.
—L.S. Bossing

A lesson plan is actually a plan of action. It therefore includes the working philosophy of the teacher, her knowledge of philosophy, her information about and understanding her pupils, her comprehension of the objectives of education, her knowledge of the material to be taught and her ability to utilize effective method.
—Lester

Purposes of Lesson Plan

- It serves as check on unplanned curriculum.
- It helps the teacher in effective teaching.
- It demands adequate consideration of goals and objectives, the selection of subject matter, the selection of teaching-learning methods, the planning of activities and the planning of evaluation devices.
- It helps the teacher to keep on track.
- It helps the teacher to carry out the teaching activity in a systematic and orderly fashion.
- It provides confidence and self-reliance to the teacher.

Principles of Lesson Planning

- It is to be used as guide and not a rule of thumb.
- The teacher should have mastery of and adequate training in the topic which the subject matter has been selected for a certain lesson.
- The teacher must be well versed with new methods and techniques of teaching nursing.
- The teacher must organize her matter in a psychological manner rather than a logical manner.
- Different teaching-learning methods should be applied to avoid monotony in the class.
- The teacher must ensure an active participation from the students in her class.

Steps for the Preparation of Lesson Plan

- **Preparation or introduction:** Exploration of the students knowledge which helps to lead them onto the lesson. The teacher has to prepare the students to receive the new knowledge. Test of previous knowledge and introduction of new topic is done.

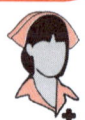

- ❏ **Presentation:** Aim of the lesson should be clearly stated before the presentation of the subject matter, which helps both the teacher and the students to have a common pursuit.
- ❏ **Comparison or association**: Quote examples, associate facts with exam, so the learners can understand very easily and arrive at generalization on their own.
- ❏ **Generalization**: It involves reflective thinking. The knowledge which will be presented by the teachers, should be thought provoking, innovating and simulating to assist the students to generalize the situation.
- ❏ **Application:** The students make use of knowledge acquire in and at the same time tests the validity of the generalization arrived at the students.
- ❏ **Recapitulation:** Teacher has to ask suitable, stimulated and pivotal questions to the students on the topic.

Prerequisites for Making Good Lesson Plan

Teacher must have:
- ❏ Good knowledge about the student's interest, traits and abilities
- ❏ Mastery over the subject matter
- ❏ Principles of teaching and learning
- ❏ Awareness of individual differences among students
- ❏ The knowledge of the students about the topic what they already possesses
- ❏ Adequate training in the topic
- ❏ Organization of material in a psychological and logical fashion
- ❏ Fully conversant with new methods and techniques of teaching the subject
- ❏ Ensure active pupil participation.

Development of a Lesson Plan

- ❏ Lesson plan should act as a guide. It should create a sense of assurance for the teacher.
- ❏ Teacher must be master of lesson plan.
- ❏ Plan should be used as a basis for continuous growth and development.
  - ▪ The teacher should change the lesson plan according to learning situation, need and ability of students.
- ❏ Lesson plan should have special work for the students who are in need of it.
- ❏ If the teacher has an air of confidence, approaches the class positively, speaks in a natural, conversational tone, asks questions in an easy manner, creates immediate interest by means of a forcible introduction, she should use all motivational, techniques.

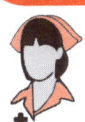

Format of a Lesson Plan

Title of the course   : _____

Unit   : _____

Topic   : _____

Name of the teacher   : _____

Duration   : _____

Date and time   : _____

Place   : _____

Class to whom teach   : _____

Number of students   : _____

Method of teaching   : _____

Audio-visual aids   : _____

- ❑ Previous knowledge/background of trainees/students
- ❑ Student teacher objectives
- ❑ General objectives
- ❑ Specific objectives

S. No	Time	Specific objectives	Content	Teaching-learning activity	Evaluation

TEACHING RESPONSIBILITIES OF A NURSE

A nurse is a teacher in so many ways. She is a teacher for her patients while giving them health education. The problems and the needs of nursing students are similar to those of all adolescents, in addition to those arising out the environment of the school of nursing. The student brings to the school her own inner life, feelings and difficulties. If the teacher guides successfully the learning activities of the nursing student, the latter may become the woman of sound judgment intellectually and morally enlightened and equipped to fulfill the nursing roles, functions and activities for which she is being prepared. She must know the student, the ways she learns about her problems.

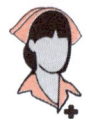

Teacher of Nursing

Ryan in his extensive work on the characteristics of teacher identified three types:
1. The warm, friendly, understanding teacher
2. The responsible, business like, systematic teacher
3. The stimulating, imaginative, creative teacher

Studies on teachers bring to mind three popular stereotypes of teachers:
1. The ever-loving
2. The tyrant
3. The rebel

A great number of teachers are good teachers in the sense that they are conscientious and devoted to teaching and students. Teaching involves communication between teacher and the taught, when each exerts a force and impact on every teaching and learning situation.

Teaching Responsibilities

The functional roles of the teacher in a school of nursing are varied and complex. They cannot be defined precisely. Teaching is never mastered, its foundations of knowledge keep on growing, and new demands and responsibilities are being constantly added.

Functional role for a teacher of nursing can be grouped into three categories:
1. Instructional
2. Faculty
3. Individual roles

Instructional Roles

- Planning and organizing courses, that is selecting objectives, substantive content, teaching and learning activities.
- Creating and maintaining congenial group climate so as to encourage and enhance learning and develop self-discipline.
- Preparing and adapting instructional material suited to the varying needs, interests and abilities of the students.
- Motivating and encouraging students to pursue learning activities which would result in their acceptance of responsibility for their own learning.

Teaching involves a series of activities as follows:
- Supplying information
- Explaining and interpreting
- Demonstrating or explaining a procedure
- Serving as a resource person
- Supervising student's performance in the classroom, laboratory, etc.
- Evaluating all the planned learning.

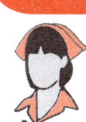

Faculty Roles

The role of a teacher as faculty member varies with the size, the control and the complexity of the institution. A faculty member may play many roles such as:

- ❏ Chairperson, secretary or member of one or more committees.
- ❏ Counselor of students in academic and nonacademic matters.
- ❏ A researcher.
- ❏ A resource person to groups outside the institution, other schools health agencies, etc.
- ❏ A representative to professional nursing organizations and other agencies for her faculty or for the institution.
- ❏ A public relation agent interpreting the objectives and the policies of her institution and helping in recruitment, etc.

Individual Roles

The teacher as an individual plays a personal role as a member of the family, a community and a citizen.

The function of the teacher range over a wide variety of activities. Preparations to assume these the teacher in a basic nursing school requires broad educational and professional training and specialized preparations in the particular field in which the teacher plans to teach, with adequate related experience in the area.

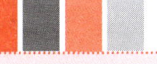 **ASSESS YOURSELF**

1. Give details of chief aspects of teaching-learning process.
2. What are the basic principles of teaching?
3. Write maxims of teaching.
4. Define learning. What are the characteristics of learning?
5. Define lesson plan, purposes of lesson plan and principles of lesson plan.
6. What are the responsibilities of a nurse as a teacher?

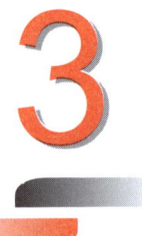

Methods of Teaching

Learning Objectives

 To narrate the methods of teaching.

To describe the clinical teaching methods.

Key Terms

- **Encompasses:** Surround and have or hold within, cause to take place.
- **Inspiration:** The action or power of moving the intellect or emotions.
- **Discovery:** Act of discovering.

INTRODUCTION

Teaching is a combination of art and science. The procedural dimension in the educative process that refers to the methods and techniques used by the teachers and learners. Every teacher has his own method of teaching and it is devised just to make the students understand.

Teacher has the only aim to educate the student and make the student understand the subject matter arranged for curriculum.

DEFINITIONS

❑ The method of teaching in which approaches most likely to the method of investigation.

—Burke

❑ A device implies the internal mode or form with teaching may take from time to time.

❑ Teaching method is the stimulation, guidance direction and encouragement of learning.

—Burton

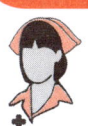

MEANING

Teaching in nursing encompasses both cognitive and artistic aspects. Art in teaching is necessary and can be developed, but this art is difficult and elusive. It is made up of moral, intellectual and aesthetic elements and of several technical skills involving operations with ideas and people.

Learning maybe stimulated and guided in various ways for different ends.

All the students have different ways of absorbing information and demonstrating their knowledge. Teacher use techniques which cater to multiple learning styles to help students retain information and strengthen understanding. A variety of methods are used to ensure that all students have equal opportunities to learn. So, the teacher has to choose the methods very carefully. There are some principles for the selection of teaching and learning methods.

PRINCIPLES FOR SELECTION OF TEACHING AND LEARNING METHODS

- ❑ The objectives and content of course
- ❑ The capacity of the student
- ❑ Accord with sound psychological principles
- ❑ Teacher's personality and capitalizes on her special assets
- ❑ Should use creativity.

OBJECTIVES

- ❑ The teaching should arise the love for work in students
- ❑ The capability of the students should be utilized to inculcate the desire to do work
- ❑ Teaching must generate the capacity for thinking in students
- ❑ Students interest should be expanded
- ❑ Provides opportunities to students to apply practically the knowledge and skill acquired by them.

CLASSIFICATION

Methods of teaching can be classified as follows:

- ❑ **Inspirational methods:** Very high activities on the part of teacher are the basis of this methods, e.g. micro teaching.
- ❑ **Expository methods:** Cognitive emphasis is high, while student activity and emphasis on experience is low, e.g. lecture method.
- ❑ **Natural learning methods:** Learning in a natural way, e.g. fields.
- ❑ **Individualized methods:** Main emphasis is that each learner should learn at its own pace by itself, e.g. self-study, computer-oriented instruction.
- ❑ **Encounter methods:** Provides experience through confrontation or through encounter effective for change in basic behavioral pattern and developing new ways of looking things, e.g. role play, simulation.

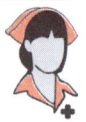

❑ **Discovery methods:** These methods are high on all dimensions like learner activity, experience, experimentation by the learner and cognitive understanding, e.g. problem solving technique.

❑ **Group methods:** For example, project method, socialized classroom method.

Let us discuss these teaching methods in an expanded form.

LECTURE METHOD

This method is also known as chalk and talk method. A lecture may be defined as carefully prepared oral presentation of facts, organized thoughts and ideas through teacher. Usually the students do not converse with the teacher. They might ask a few questions, but these are for the sake of clarification, not for the sake of discussion.

Definition

Presentation of the contents by the teacher to the students is usually accompanied by some type of visual aid or handouts.

Purpose of Lecture Method

In many circumstances, the lecture method may be the only appropriate one, for making available to large classes, the instructional services of an expert teaching and/or scholar. The lecture should not be a representation of exactly what is in the textbook neither in the assigned reading nor should it be completely unrelated to student's reading. The lecture should illuminate, supplement and reinforce the topic being studied. A lecture properly prepared and delivered can have an organizing or integrating function. The teacher may communicate through her lecture such relative intangible as enthusiasm for a subject, tolerance or respect for ideas, worthwhile of intellectual values in general, by means of her manner, her mode of presentation and her materials.

Preparation of a Lecture

The goal of lecturing is communication and it is likely to be more effective if it is prepared before. The lecture should have a central theme carried to be completion in each delivery. It should contain sequence of ideas kept relatively simple with headings and subheadings.

The lecture with too many points has no point at all. The lecture should be written in outline form. The amount of details will vary with the teacher's experience in lecturing and his/her knowledge of the subject.

Technique of the Lecture

❑ The lecture is viewed not only as a means of presenting information but also as a method of effective learning. It requires the teacher not only to talk but to work with the students. This means that the teacher establishes contact with the student quickly and paces her delivery to the capacity of her students to follow her lecture, making allowances for note-taking. She will make sure that the important points in her lecture are made clear before proceeding to the next point. There are some guidelines which should be followed for a good lecture delivering.

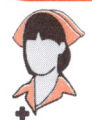

- ❑ **Rapport:** The teacher should at the outset of the lecture try to establish rapport with her students by exchanging with them about some event at the school, by beginning the lecture with a review of previous lectures and through questions.
- ❑ **Voice:** The lecture should be presented in a clear natural tone of the voice.
- ❑ **Gesture:** Whatever gesture the lecturer used should be spontaneous and animated and a part of natural style of the individual.
- ❑ **Eye contact:** The lecture should be addressed not only with voice but with eyes also.
- ❑ **Lecture outline and students notes:** The lecture should be prepared and delivered in several blocks and units. Each unit presentable is not more than fifteen minutes duration of continuous talk. The lecture should be presented from written notes but should not be read. The lecture should be delivered on the assumption that the students have completed the reading assignments and are prepared. Before beginning her lectures, the teacher will have her entire course prepared.

Advantages

- ❑ Lecture method is a method which is straight forward way and can give knowledge quickly to the students.
- ❑ Teacher is physically present in the class.
- ❑ It can cover a large group of students.
- ❑ Presence of teacher gives security feeling to the students.
- ❑ It helps in apparent saving of time and resources.
- ❑ Multiple resource persons, knowledge and with different points of view can interact with students.
- ❑ A large number of students can be accommodated at one time.
- ❑ Lecture contains experience which inspires.
- ❑ It stimulates thinking to open discussion.

Disadvantages and Limitations

- ❑ Decrease student's involvement in learning when content is readily available and easy to understand.
- ❑ This method creates difficulty who are weak in taking notes and have trouble in understanding what they should remember from lectures.
- ❑ Keeps the students in a passive situation.
- ❑ Asking of questions or queries during lecture is difficult.
- ❑ The lecture expert may not be a good teacher.
- ❑ May have high cost in preparation and development of visual aid.
- ❑ Learning is difficult to gauge.
- ❑ Communication is one way.

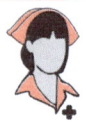

DEMONSTRATION METHOD

It is a physically display of the form, outline or substance of object or events for the purpose of increasing knowledge of such objects or events. As a rule, courses of education use demonstration in the form of demonstration-lecture. In nursing education, it is used for clinics, conference, laboratory classes, symposia, autopsies and teaching of health to the patients. The demonstration method therefore, of utmost importance in the teaching of nursing. The demonstration method teaches by exhibition and explanation.

Guidelines for Good Demonstration

- The demonstrator or teacher should plan and rehearsal beforehand.
- The demonstration, equipment and teacher should be visible to the whole class.
- Class or demonstration area should have a good physical setup.
- All equipment should be assembled and pretested before the demonstration takes place. This saves time and ensures that the apparatus will be in good state.
- The purpose and objectives of the demonstration should be clear to the students before starting demonstration.
- Active participation of the students is mandatory.
- The unnecessarily linger on of the demonstration should be avoided.
- The interest of the students should be continued.
- The running comments should be continuing during the demonstration.
- The prompt practice and return demonstration to evolve the level of understanding of the students should be taken.

Advantages

- Presence of teacher gives a feeling of security to the students.
- It activates several senses and visibly showing a process often helps in retention.
- Develops quality of observation and provide observational learning.
- Correlates theory and practical.
- Ensure closer contact with concrete problems.
- Facilitates the acquisition of practical, intellectual and communication skills.
- Presents reality, not substitutes.
- Enables logical step by step presentation.
- It attention catching.
- Demonstration is the right way of doing a complex task.
- Presented facing the audience.
- Makes it possible to clear queries.
- Limits damages to equipment and material when students do practical work afterwards.
- Helps teacher to evaluate the student's response.
- Facilitates return demonstration.

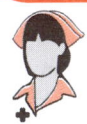

Disadvantages

- Number of students is limited
- Keeps the students in a passive situation
- Offers little possibility of checking the learning process
- Does not allow for individual pieces of learning
- High cost in personnel and time
- Difficulty in repeating demonstration in order to acquire competence.

DISCUSSION METHOD

Discussion is a democratic method of teaching which may be used:

- For teaching a particular subject
- To supplement a lecture
- In connection with an observation visit or case presentation
- For a penal discussion.

General Principles of Discussion

The general principles related to the organization of discussion are as follows:

- There should be clearly defined objectives which are understood by all the participants.
- There should be one leader to guide and co-ordinate the proceedings.
- The main points in the discussion should be recorded as it is going on either on blackboard or by a recorder elected by the group.
- Every person should feel free to participate.
- Timid persons should be encouraged to contribute.
- All points of view should be fairly considered.
- Discussion should be kept to the point.
- The discussion should be properly closed with a report, decision, recommendation or summing up of the matters discussed.
- The members of the group should come to the discussion with a basic knowledge of the topic to be discussed.

Forms of Discussion (Fig. 1)

Class Discussion

The teacher may select the discussion method for teaching a particular topic, with the whole class participating as one group. This can be managed quite efficiently if the class is not too large. The teacher acting as leader, will present the topic guide and direct the discussion, note the main points on the blackboard and assist the group summing up. This method is useful when the students have a prior knowledge of the subject. It can serve as a learning experience for students on how to conduct discussion.

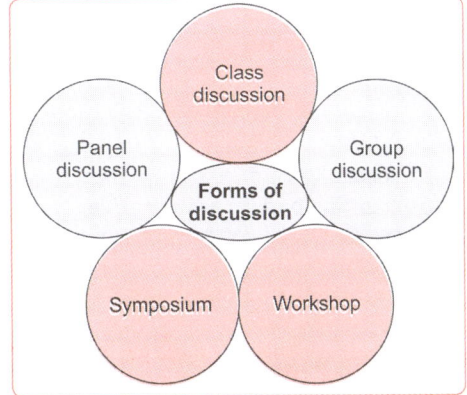

Fig. 1: Forms of discussion

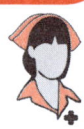

Advantages

- ❏ Pools ideas and experiences from group.
- ❏ Effective after a presentation, film or experience that needs to be analyzed.
- ❏ Allows everyone to participate in an active process.

Disadvantages

- ❏ Not practicable with more than 20 people
- ❏ Few people can dominate
- ❏ Others may not participate
- ❏ Can get off the track.

Panel Discussion

This method was originated by "Professor Harry Allen Overstreet. Panel is a discussion in which 4–8 persons who are qualified about the topic carry on a conversation in front of audience. The panel method has one chairperson/chairman, the members of the panel and audience. They all sits in a semicircle facing the audience. The chairman starts the meeting, introduces the topic to be discussed. There is no specific agenda, no order of speaking and no set speeches. It is an extremely effected method of teaching, provided it is properly planned and guided.

Advantages

- ❏ Allows experts to present different opinions.
- ❏ Can provoke better discussion than one-person discussion.
- ❏ Frequent change of speaker keeps attention from lagging.

Disadvantages

- ❏ Experts may not be good speakers.
- ❏ Personalities may over shadow contents.
- ❏ Subjects may not in logical order.

Group Discussion

A group discussion is teaching and sharing the ideas with a group of students or people. This method is considered as very effective method of education especially in health-related communication. It is a method which allows the free flow of ideas and help the members a wide range of interaction.

The ideal group for group discussion should be 6–12 members. The participants should sit in a circular sitting pattern as they all can see each other. A group leader should be selected who initiates the discussion and controls the discussion. The chairman or leader also sums up the discussion in the net. Among the group one person should act as recorder who records all the discussion so that in the end of the discussion reports can be written. Some rules should be followed by the members which are as follows:

- ❏ Experts should put their ideas clearly and concisely.
- ❏ Members should be good listeners also they should listen what others say.

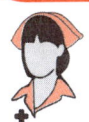

- Be brief, do not monopolize the discussion.
- Indulge in friendly disagreement.
- Active participation by all the members is must. It should be with relevant remarks. No personal remarks should be given.
- Accept criticism gracefully.
- Help to reach conclusion.
- Keep contact on the voice and gestures.

Advantages

- It allows the learners to be in control, in respect of pace, content and focus.
- It provides opportunities to the learner to express themselves.
- It allows learner to validate their knowledge and skills.
- It permits learners to clarify, reflect and reconfigure their experience.
- It helps in promoting a sense of belonging in a group.
- It can be empowering if learners realize their own ability for critical thinking and change through this medium.

Disadvantages

- It requires facilitation and if facilitation is poor then the process is vitiated.
- Requires more space than lecture.
- Time consuming.
- It is difficult to monitor the progress of many small groups.
- When dominant members are not controlled it can affect the participation of other members of the group.

Symposium

It is a method of group discussion in which two or more persons under the direction of chairman present separate speeches which give several aspects of one question. Its purpose is to investigate a problem from several points of view. The purpose is not to give a series of arguments in debate. The symposium generally consists of a set of programs prepared speeches followed by audience discussion. The procedure is like that of a straight lecture forum, except that several people present speeches representing different approaches to the same problem. The symposium method generally presents a wider basis for discussion than the lecture method, because it presents a topic from several points of view. It has a greater organization than other discussion methods because of the set of speeches prepared beforehand.

Advantages

- It gives wider basis for discussion, because it presents the topic from several points of view.
- It has a greater impact to pre-prepared speeches.

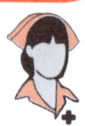

Disadvantages

- ❑ Lack of time usually one speaker gets 10–15 minutes only.
- ❑ Student's participation is very-very less.
- ❑ Audience participation is limited to one or two questions only.

Workshop

Definition

A workshop is the work of a group of individuals who work together towards the solution of problems in a given subject matter field during a specific period of time. The group members of the workshop select the objectives them self.

Principles

- ❑ To increase the participants or group members motivation allow the members to prepare and select the objectives.
- ❑ An active role should be given to the group members to make teaching more effective.
- ❑ The participants should have the regular opportunities to see and work which is learned in workshop.
- ❑ Person attitude towards other people.
- ❑ To learn better human relationship.
- ❑ Every individual has worth, and has a contribution make common goods.
- ❑ The most crucial learning at any given time has to do with the individual's current problems.
- ❑ Cooperation is a technique and as a way of life which is superior to competition, is primary factor to be allowed.

Working Method of a Workshop (Flow chart 1)

The working method of a workshop follows the following steps which are self-explanatory and helps in learning:

- ❑ After organizing a workshop, we have to send thanks letter to the speaker and prepare the report of the workshop with minutes of workshop and response of program evaluation.

Outcome of a Workshop

It widens specific knowledge, profession and personal growth. It increases friendships, team spirit and human relations.

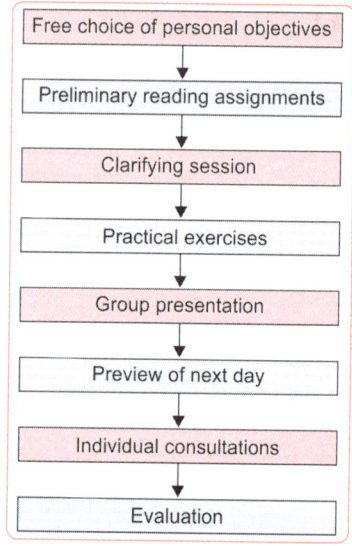

Flow chart 1: Working method of a workshop

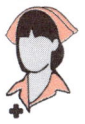

CLINICAL TEACHING METHOD

Clinical teaching as name indicates is a teaching method in the clinical area. It is vital and irreplaceable component in preparing students for the reality of their professional role. In nursing the curriculum is such that it correlates the subject matter learned in ideal situation to the real situation. The clinical instructor organizes the clinical experiences and the student nurse learns the bedside nursing from the senior nursing professional, senior students is real field situations. Clinical instruction is directly concerned with teaching students about the care of clients.

In clinical area, the student nurse will learn technical skills, by doing the activity and practicing their theoretical knowledge into practice. The students will practice and gain skills, based on scientific principles. The teaching methods will improve the qualitative care, students can practice and provide good quality care. Various clinical teaching methods are listed as follows:

❑ Client family centered method
❑ Observation:
  ▪ Participant
  ▪ Nonparticipant
❑ Conferences
  ▪ Clinical conference
  ▪ Individual conference
  ▪ Group conference
  ▪ Staff conference
  ▪ Nursing case conference
  ▪ Team conference
❑ Bedside clinics
❑ Nursing rounds and medical rounds
❑ Demonstration and re-demonstration of procedures
❑ Ward teaching
❑ Ward class
❑ Ward clinic
❑ Care study/case presentation
❑ Group discussion
❑ Brain storming method
❑ Process recording
❑ Laboratory method
❑ Incidental and planned health talks
❑ Nursing case study
❑ Organizing exhibition
❑ Incidental teaching
❑ Problem solving ring method
❑ Research projects

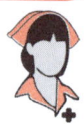

From these all we will discuss about the following methods in detail:

- ❑ Case method
- ❑ Bedside clinics
- ❑ Nursing rounds
- ❑ Nursing conference
- ❑ Process recording

CASE METHOD

The case method of teaching and learning is often used with group discussion. It has been used extensively as a prime method of teaching in nursing than any other methods.

Case methods are used in three forms. They are as follows:

1. **Case study:** It is a method to study a case in depth. A specific patent/client is assigned to the student for 4 to 5 days. She has to give comprehensive care to the patient and prepare a case study with history of patient and the case of patient. She compares the problems, solutions with the text. The student presents the case before the group and general discussion about the patient is done.

2. **Case analysis method:** Case analysis method of teaching focus on a central situation which requires some decision or solution. It presents a concrete case for analysis and discussion by a group of students under the leadership of clinical instructor. Adequate information is presented to the students for them to make judgments on a problem or situation.

   The main objective of the case analysis method of teaching is that student nurses able to identify the problem them self and able to handle the situation with the needed skills. They should extend the ability to utilize date from experience as a test of validity of the ideas already obtained with flexibility to revise goals and procedures which the need arises.

3. **Case incident method/techniques:** Case incident method is a modified type of the case analysis method organized by the Paul and Faith Pigers. A critical incident technique which requires immediate decision and action is taken from a case and presented to the students for their analysis and decision.

   No background information is given to them regarding the details of the incident at the time, it is presented. The instructor will have the facts about the case, can be given as requested by the students.

The Pigers, suggests the five-phase process for the valuable use of case incident method:

Phase I   : The Incidence—Selected patient/Situation

Phase II   : Getting the facts—From the discussion and observation

Phase III : Determining the source of problem and the consequences

Phase IV : Stating decisions and reasons for decision by individual students

Phase V   : Identifying the major decisions and issues raised by the individual students through group discussion.

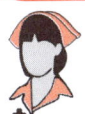

BEDSIDE CLINICS

Bedside clinics always entail the presence of the patient. Either the group visits bedside or the patient is brought to the conference room.

Forms of Bedside Clinics

❑ Clinics may be given by the doctor in which case symptoms, medical therapy and emphasized.
❑ Nursing clinics are conducted by head nurse or clinical instructor.

Preparation for Nursing Clinics

Nurses who are to present patients in a bedside clinic should know long enough in advance to be able to make necessary preparation. The amount of time required depends upon nurse's experience, in this type of teaching his/her knowledge of the patient's history and nursing care. No one should be asked to present a patient on whom he/she had not got an opportunity to read all data related to patient and patient care. If he/she is used to organizing such material, he/she may require one-hour time and if not he/she should require several days to prepare and be given whatever assistance he/she need.

Method of Conducting Nursing Bedside Clinics

In nursing clinic, the patient's medical history and therapy are discussed briefly. The problems of patient identified are described and emphasis is placed on his nursing care involving all dimensions of health.

❑ Patients with typical rather than unusual conditions should be selected for clinics. The dramatic and atypical condition may leave the students with erroneous impressions. Perhaps, when nurse has the opportunity to observe and converse with the patient related to his health and illness, he/she would remember the nursing measures used to meet his needs better.
❑ The group in attendance at the clinic should be small enough to gather around the bed in an informal way, in order to make the patient at ease.
❑ Patient in not required to remain the whole discussion. Before the patient bought for discussion, one should describe about the profile of patient, history of medical illness with biographical information. This should be extended to medical history and therapy as they relate to nursing care.
❑ Head nurse/clinical instructor may lead the discussion. They will point out the group before the arrival of the patient for the observation that has to be made accurately on the patients.
❑ Then the patient is brought to the discussion since many points may be clarified and questions may be raised. When the patient is no longer needed, he/she is returned to the unit.
❑ Clinic may last for 30 minutes but if any specialist is asked to participate time may be extended.
❑ In the last, following the clinic, the head nurse/clinical instructor should evaluate the effectiveness of presentation.

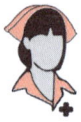

NURSING ROUNDS

A small group of the staff members, not more than five and a leader and a teacher visit, the bedside of clients. Nursing superintendents, ward sisters taking rounds of the hospital wards. It helps the nursing members know about all the patients in the wards, their problems and ways of solving. It is an extension of the clinic method.

Procedure for Conducting Nursing Rounds

❑ Students have to be given information about ward rounds, so that, it will help them, to prepare themselves for the learner experience.

❑ Students will be following nursing rounds. The clinical instructor will stop briefly at the bedside of each patient for a short discussion of the most significant nursing problem.

❑ The instructor may instruct any nurse in the group to tell what she knows about the client and his nursing care.

❑ The student who is taking care of the patient for a week or so, he/she has to present the case of the total group of the students so that all the students will be aware about the case and its total condition. If any cardinal manifestations are identified, with the client's permission they can demonstrate to the total group. The presentation of the background information is followed by additions and suggestions from the group.

❑ Case presentation should be short and relate only to problem or situation of immediate interest.

❑ The contents to be discussed in nursing rounds carefully selected, well organized clearly and interestingly presented for each client only 3–4 minutes have to be spent.

Purpose of Nursing Rounds

The purpose of nursing rounds is to expose learners to more and more nursing situations and to encourage them to consult with each other in planning and evaluating nursing care. Nursing rounds provide many opportunities to apply classroom theory to patient situations and to compare and contrast the patient care.

Post clinical conference becomes more meaningful when students have met many or all the patients being discussed.

The practice of nursing rounds is a teaching strategy that uses bedside for direct and puposeful activities.

Rounds can afford an excellent opportunity for the exchange of ideas about patient care situation.

Disadvantages

❑ Requires careful planning.

❑ A small group of students can be taken at a time.

❑ Can cause discomfort to patient.

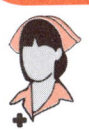

NURSING CONFERENCE

Although nursing care conferences may be conducted in many different ways. It is essentially the same method of teaching as bedside clinic. In nursing care conference, the patient is usually not present for any part of the class. This may be the method of choice when the entire group is well known with patient and would have nothing new to learn from going to see him.

Individual Conference

Individual conference is described as conversation with purpose. The specific purpose in the interview is to obtain facts or to provide information. The individual conference can be used by the clinical instructor to clarify class material, to supplement instructions to explain answers to questions of individual students which do not concern the entire class. Individual conference facilitates nursing students to understand the relationship between class contents of course and the application problems of nursing practice and patient care.

Group Conference

Group conference is the act of consulting together, any coming together of two or more individuals in a formal meeting for the purpose of giving or exchanging ideas. It involves a two-way flow of conversation.

The main purpose of group conference is to set objectives and criteria for nursing care. This helps in planning methods for improving care and solves problems which interfere with good nursing care. It evaluates results of efforts.

Time for Conference

Conference may be held at any period of the day when the members (staff/students etc.) are free to attend. It should be planned on the same hours weekly so that the members mark themselves free at that hour.

Place for Conference

The four things should be kept in mind while considering the place of conference.

1. Patients must not be able to listen any part of the discussion.
2. Seating arrangements are essential.
3. Patient's signals must register in conference room unless some member of the staff remains away from the meeting to care for patients.
4. The place for conference should be one where interruption will be minimal.

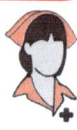

PROCESS RECORDING

It is a learning tool which aids a student to develop observation and communication skills.

Definitions

A verbatim account of a visit for purpose of bringing out the interplay between the nurse and the patient in relation to the objectives of visit.   —*Walker*

An exact written report of the conversation between nurse and the patient during the time they were together and record of the nurse's feeling about what was going on at the time and as far as possible, how the patient said what he did.   —*Hudson*

Purpose

❑ Guide the students in the development of self-awareness of own behaviors—verbal and non-verbal on a patient.

❑ Encourage students to use variety of strategies to accomplish the stated communication goal.

❑ Enable students to become more objective in the processing of patient messages.

❑ Create opportunity for students to propose alternative responses to patient messages for faculty feedback.

❑ Provide the student with the comparative record of own progress in the development of communication skills.

❑ Help the teacher to gain understanding of student's progress in the ability towards therapeutic communication.

The process recording may be used as data collection instrument for the following three purposes also

1. As a teaching tool.
2. As a self-evaluation tool.
3. As a therapeutic tool.

Phases

❑ **Preparing the student for process recording:** The teacher must help the student to define clearly the objectives to be accomplished regarding nurse-patient interactions.

❑ **Recording nurse-patient interactions:**
   ▪ The exact report of the patient-nurse conversation.
   ▪ The student's conscious feelings and her interpretation of the patient's feelings.
   ▪ Analysis for meanings and clues to patient's needs.
   ▪ The instructor's and the student's evaluation of total process recording experience.

❑ **Evaluating the nurse-patient interactions:**
  ■ After the interaction, data have been collected by the student, the teacher and student have to analysis the recordings based on objectives
  ■ Self-evaluation by the student to develop a deeper understanding of her own behavior and the effect of her behavior on others.
  ■ Develops keener insight into the behavior of the patient.

Advantages

❑ Helps student to have an objective look of his/her own communication skills.
❑ Provides teacher with an accurate account of the student's clinical learning experience.
❑ Assists the teacher to explore the areas where students require improvement or refine in communication skills.

Disadvantages

❑ Lengthy involvement of time in teaching and implementing this tool.
❑ It cannot record all non-verbal causes like mannerisms, time or impressions well.

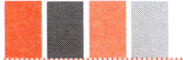 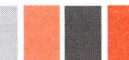

ASSESS YOURSELF

1. Define methods of teaching and classify them.
2. Enlist methods of teaching and describe in detail any two of them.
3. Explain nursing conference in details.

Notes

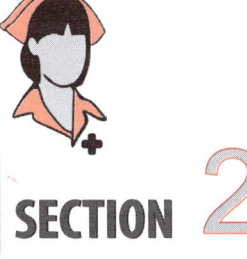

SECTION 2

INTRODUCTION TO RESEARCH

- ➲ Introduction

- ➲ Research Process

- ➲ Research Approaches/Research Design

- ➲ Data Collection Process

- ➲ Analysis of Data

- ➲ Writing a Report

- ➲ Introduction to Statistics

- ➲ Utilization of Research Findings

Introduction

4

Research is a scientific process and a high headed word which creates fear in so many people. In fact, as it is systematic search for answers to the questions about facts and relationship between facts, it is called scientific because the results are verifiable.

Research in every field especially in nursing is demand of the day. It is necessary and has direct linkage to the progress of the field.

DEFINITION AND MEANING OF RESEARCH

The term "research" is derivative of the word 'recherché; which means, *'quest, search or pursuit'*. It may be understood as a search for truth; a search after truth; or make searches to conduct a close investigation and inquiry. The other meaning of the word research is to search again or to examine carefully. More specifically the research is a systematic inquiry.

American Public Health Association (APHA) in 1956 defines the research as:

Research is the studying of problems in pursuit of a definite objective through employing precise methods, with due considerations to the adequate control factors other than the variables under investigation and followed by analysis according to statistical procedure.

❑ Research in an abstract and selection from an infinite variety of possible things that one might study.

—Gowin and Millman 1969

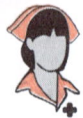

- ❑ Research essentially is a problem-solving process, a systematic intensive study directed towards full scientific knowledge of the subject studied.   —*French Ruth M 1968*
- ❑ Research is a careful enquiry or examination, is seeking facts or principles, a diligent investigation to ascertain something.   —*Clifford Woody*
- ❑ Research is in the way of dealing with ideas. It is nothing more than, that, this and it is nothing.   —*Barnes*
- ❑ Research is process systematically searches for new facts and relationships.   —*Notter*

STEPS IN SCIENTIFIC METHOD

Science is a unified body of systematized knowledge concerned with specific subject matter obtained by establishing and organizing facts, principles and methods. A goal of science is to develop theories that can describe, explain and predict phenomena and that can ultimately be used to control phenomena. Phenomenas are the facts or events known through senses rather than by thought or intuition and that can be scientifically described. Research is scientific endeavor. It involves scientific method. Scientific method is systematic step-by-step procedure following the logical processes of reasoning. Scientific method is a means of gaining knowledge of the universe.

Simply stated, scientific research, whether basic or applied, involves the following steps:

- ❑ Identifying the problem, state it clearly, and delimiting it to a manageable research question.
- ❑ Collecting essential facts pertaining to the problem. This includes reviewing the literature, validating the significance of the problem, and selecting or developing theories to explain the problem and to suggest its solution.
- ❑ Formulate a prediction of an expected outcome.
- ❑ Setting up a suitable design or method for the study.
- ❑ Collecting the essential data required for answering the research questions.
- ❑ Analyzing the findings of the research.
- ❑ Communicate the findings of the research study.

Limitations of Scientific Method

- ❑ Moral and ethical problems
- ❑ Human complexity
- ❑ Measurement problems
- ❑ External variables control problems.

NURSING RESEARCH

The main goal of nursing is to provide ultimate and high-quality care to the patients. Research is needed to evaluate the effectiveness of nursing treatment modalities, traditional ways, impact of nursing care on the health of the people, or to test theories. In order to meet the social challenges, tremendous changes, needs, nursing practices must be research based.

Nursing research is defined as the application of scientific inquiry to the phenomena of concern to nursing. Nursing research seeks to find, new knowledge that can eventually be applied in providing nursing care to patients. Nursing research develops knowledge about health and

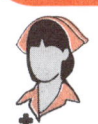

promotion of health over the full life span, care of person with health problems and disabilities to respond effectively to actual or potential health problems.
(Commission of Nursing Research, American Nurses Association, 1981)

Nursing research is a way to identify new knowledge, improve professional education and practices and use of resources effectively.
(International Council of Nurses, 1986)

Need and Purposes of Nursing Research

To go ahead and to meet the new challenges of the profession research is must. Nurses engage in research for number of reasons. In addition to establish a scientific base of knowledge for profession the systematic accrual of nursing information enables nurses to better define the nursing parameters and develop theoretical framework for clinical practices and enhance the professional skills for nurses. Research is a fundamental essential prerequisite for any profession. The specific purpose of nursing research includes identification, description, exploration, explanation, prediction and control of facts. Therefore, nursing research enables nurses in the following ways:

- Develop, refine and extend the scientific base of knowledge, which is required for quality nursing care, education and administration.
- Filling the gaps in the knowledge and practice.
- Fostering a commitment accountability to clientele.
- To molding the attitudes and intellectual competence and technical skills.
- Providing basis for professionalism and professional accountability.
- To identify the role of nurse in changing society.
- Discovering new measures, helping to take prompt decisions in nursing practices and administration.
- To improve the standards of nursing education.
- Refining existing theories and discovering new theories.

Characteristics of Good Research

Research employs scientific methods. Good research is systematic, logical, empirical, and also replicable. A good research must satisfy the following criteria:

- A research should be conducted in an orderly and systematic process
- Research must be based on current professional issues
- Research should begin with clearly defined purpose
- Research should emphasize to develop, refine and expand professional knowledge
- It should be directed towards development or testing theories
- A research is, finding solution of problem
- A research always strives to develop empirical evidences
- It should strive to collect first-hand information/data
- A good research emphasizes on objective and logical research process
- Generate findings to refine and improve professional practices can be the aim of a good research
- A good research always employs the most appropriate and suitable methodology

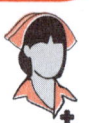

- ❑ A good research is conducted on a representative sample
- ❑ Research should be conducted through appropriate use of methods and tools of data collection
- ❑ A good research should be very carefully recorded and reported
- ❑ Research requires courage
- ❑ Patience and endurance are the foundation of good research
- ❑ A research cannot be considered good until the information generated is adequately disseminated to its users, therefore a good research activity strives to communicate findings as widely as possible.

Importance of Nursing Research

Research is a fundamental and essential prerequisite for any profession. As nursing is a budding profession the need and importance of the nursing research is quite significant.

- ❑ It helps to develop, refine and extend the scientific base of knowledge, which is required for quality nursing care, education and administration
- ❑ It enhances the body of professional knowledge in nursing
- ❑ Research is the foundation for evidence-based nursing
- ❑ It expands the knowledge and continues the growth of profession
- ❑ Seek new truths and add to find the knowledge and discipline
- ❑ Fills the gap between knowledge and practice
- ❑ Redirect course of action and evaluate policies
- ❑ Define parameters of nursing which will help to identify the boundaries of nursing profession
- ❑ Helps to develop and define theories, models and principles of nursing
- ❑ It helps to solve the problems and questions related to nursing education and nursing administration
- ❑ It discovers new facts about known phenomena
- ❑ It improves the existing technique and develops new instruments or procedures
- ❑ It shows the pathway of action of known substances.

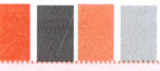 **ASSESS YOURSELF**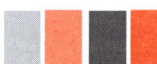

1. What do you understand by the term research?
2. Describe the steps of scientific methods of research.
3. Do you think research is a need for nursing? Explain.
4. What are the characteristics of good research?

Research Process

5

Learning Objective

 To describe the research process.

Key Terms

- **Research process:** A technique used to structure a study in systematic manner.
- **Research problem:** Refers to some difficulty which researcher experiences.

According to Talbot LA: Research is a scientific process of enquiry that involves purposeful, systematic and rigorous collection, analysis and interpretation of data to gain new knowledge. So we can say that research starts from the problem or question and ends with the generation and dissemination of an answer to that problem or question. It is a step-by-step process followed by one after another.

As qualitative and quantitative researches are not similar so there is a difference between the both of the processes.

To start with the steps of the research process we will have an overview of the both researches process in a tabular way.

❑ Steps of qualitative research process (Flow chart 1).

Flow chart 1: Steps of qualitative research process

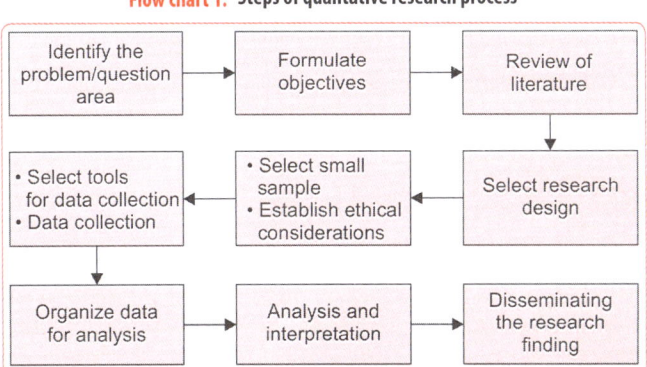

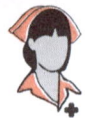

❑ Steps of quantitative research process (Flow chart 2).

Flow chart 2: Steps of quantitative research process

```
┌─────────────────┐      ┌─────────────────┐      ┌─────────────────┐
│  Formulation of │ ───▶ │  Establishing   │ ───▶ │   Review of     │
│ research problem│      │   the study     │      │   literature    │
│                 │      │   objectives    │      │                 │
└─────────────────┘      └─────────────────┘      └─────────────────┘
                                                           │
                                                           ▼
┌─────────────────┐      ┌─────────────────┐      ┌─────────────────┐
│   Selection of  │ ◀─── │  Formulating    │ ◀─── │   Developing    │
│ research design │      │   hypothesis    │      │   conceptual    │
│                 │      │                 │      │   framework     │
└─────────────────┘      └─────────────────┘      └─────────────────┘
         │
         ▼
┌─────────────────┐      ┌─────────────────┐      ┌─────────────────┐
│  Specifying the │ ───▶ │ Developing tools/│ ───▶ │    Ethical      │
│   population    │      │  techniques for │      │  considerations │
│                 │      │ data collection │      │                 │
└─────────────────┘      └─────────────────┘      └─────────────────┘
                                                           │
                                                           ▼
┌─────────────────┐      ┌─────────────────┐      ┌─────────────────┐
│ Data collection │ ◀─── │ Sample selection│ ◀─── │    Have a       │
│                 │      │                 │      │   pilot study   │
└─────────────────┘      └─────────────────┘      └─────────────────┘
         │
         ▼
┌─────────────────┐      ┌─────────────────┐
│  Analysis and   │ ───▶ │ Disseminating the│
│ interpretation of│     │    findings     │
│      data       │      │                 │
└─────────────────┘      └─────────────────┘
```

Now let us start the process step-by-step.

QUALITATIVE RESEARCH DESIGN

Advantages

Qualitative research is a systematic, interactive, subjective approach used to describe life experience and give them meaning. This is easier to conduct as compared to the quantitative research design. Phenomenological, ethnographic, grounded theory historical, case studies are the main types of the qualitative research designs.

Disadvantages

It is more time, money and energy consuming. It involves various data collection strategies and it may involve multiple sites. This study cannot be done by beginning researchers.

QUANTITATIVE RESEARCH DESIGN

Advantages

Quantitative research design can be further divided into experimental and nonexperimental studies. This type of design has precise measurements and quantification often involving rigorous and controlled designs.

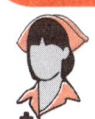

Disadvantages

This is a limited study. Sometimes artificiality may be there. Hawthorne effect may be seen.

These two qualitative and quantitative approaches have emerged in recent years to develop nursing knowledge.

STEPS OF RESEARCH PROCESS

Nursing research is systematic, logical, empirical and also replicable. The major steps in conducting research are:

❏   Identification of research problem
❏   Literature review
❏   Specifying the purpose of research
❏   Determining specific research questions
❏   Specification of a conceptual framework usually a set of hypotheses
❏   Methodology
❏   Data collection
❏   Analyzing and interpreting the data
❏   Reporting and evaluation research
❏   Communicating the research findings and recommendations.

RESEARCH PROBLEM

Statement of Research Problem

This is the first step of the research and it is most basic and most difficult phase of the research project. The problem statement typically identifies the study variables and population, and it must explicitly and unambiguously define the problem topic and provide guidelines for the expected answer.

Components of Research Problem

A problem statement generally has six components:
1.   Relevance of the study.
2.   Title of the study.
3.   Operational definitions of variables.
4.   Objectives of study.
5.   Delimitations of study.
6.   Scope and limitations of study.

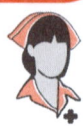

Sources of Research Problem

It is a question and an itself problem for each and every researcher that from where he/she should look for a significant and genuine research problem. Following are some of the sources from which we can have a research problem:

- ❑ Previous research
- ❑ Every day observations and experience
- ❑ Nursing literature
- ❑ Social issues
- ❑ Theories and conceptual schemes
- ❑ Ideas from external sources
- ❑ Patients/relatives feedback
- ❑ Empirical interests
- ❑ Political concerns
- ❑ Critical appraisal of literature
- ❑ Brain storming
- ❑ Consultations with experts
- ❑ Interest of professional organizations.

Criteria for Selection of a Good Research Problem

There are many factors which should be considered while finding and selecting a research problem. As an English proverb that "Right start is half work done" same is with research selection of a "good a right problem" followed by its analysis and formulation is half the research work accomplished.

For a good research problem, factors are as follows:

- ❑ **Significance to nursing profession:**
  - ▪ Nursing professionals and patients, nurses and health care fraternity will benefit from the study
  - ▪ The results will improve clinical nursing practice
  - ▪ Promotes nursing theory development or testing
  - ▪ Provides solutions of current nursing practice needs
  - ▪ Generate information to get practical implications for nursing profession
- ❑ It should be original, i.e. it should be new and unique in itself
- ❑ It should be feasible. Feasibility is an essential condition of any research project. Feasibility and research problem in reference to time, availability of subjects, facilities, equipment and money, ethical considerations should be checked. This will help to see whether the study can be conducted or not
  - ▪ **Time:** Time is one factor which should be considered for the research. Sometime unexpected delays can occur so the time limit should be set and managed very wisely.
  - ▪ **Cost:** It is a factor which basically affects the studies, the financial conditions and financial assistance should be kept in mind so that the project should be completed within the set budget.

- **Equipment and supplies:** An accurate determination of the needed equipment and supplies should be ensured before selecting the problem for research.
- **Administration and peer group support:** Administrative support is very helpful for the research projects as it gives the powerful motivational support to the work and help to cross the hurdles of the work. A climate of research is made only with the help peer group support. They give ideas and extend help.
- **Availability of subjects:** It is to consider that the subjects should be available in a sufficient number so that the person can make the conclusions for study.
- **Researcher competence and ethical considerations** should be kept for the feasibility of the research problem.

❑ **Researchable:** The problem should be solvable or researchable and should enhance relevant results.

❑ **Current:** Current issues of the profession can be considered so that results generated will be of more use.

❑ **Interesting:** A problem can only be considered good if it is in accordance with researcher field of interest. It motivates, fascinates and gives more knowledge to the researcher.

Formulation of Research Problem

Formulation of research problem is a long and complex process. It includes the following steps:

❑ Selection of research area
❑ Reviewing of literature and theories
❑ Delimiting the research topic
❑ Evaluating the research problems
❑ Formulating final statement of research problem.

Steps in formulating problem statement (Flow chart 3).

Flow chart 3: Steps in formulating problem statement

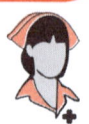

WRITING RESEARCH OBJECTIVES

To do a research, the objectives have a very important and significant place. Clearly defined objectives enlighten the way in which the researcher has to proceed. Without focused objectives, no replicable scientific finding can be expected from any type of research.

Hence, a research objective is clear concise declarative statement, which provides direction to investigate the variables.

Characteristics

The research should have the following key research objectives:

- It should be specific
- It should be measurable
- It should be attainable
- It should be realistic
- It should be time bound

So a well worded objective will be SMART.

- A research objective should have the other properties like: it should be relevant, feasible, logical observable, unequivocal and measurable.
- The objective should be such which can summarizes that what can be achieved by the research project and the study.
- The objective should specifically accomplish the researcher's hope to be achieved by the study and it include obtaining answers to research questions testing the research hypothesis.

Need

Research objectives help the researcher to:

- Focus on study
- Avoid the unnecessary finding
- The formulation of objectives organize the study in clearly defined parts
- Proper and specific objectives give directions to conduct the research.

Types

- **General objectives:** These are broad goals to be achieved. These are usually less in number.
- **Specific objectives:** These objectives are short-term and narrow in focus and systematically addressed.

  If the objectives have not been spelled out clearly, the project cannot be considered complete.

TERMS AND DEFINITIONS USED IN RESEARCH

- **Abstract:** It is clear, concise summary of a study, usually limited to 100–250 words, expressed without reference to any incident.

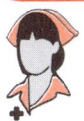

- **Action research:** A research approach in which researchers pursue action and research outcomes at the same time.
- **Adoption:** Full acceptance and implementation of an innovation in practice.
- **Accuracy:** Address the extent in which a physiological instrument measures the concept defined in the study.
- **Anonymity:** Conditions in which the subjects identity cannot be linked, even by the researcher, with his or her individual response.
- **Assumption:** Statement taken for granted or considered true, even though, they have not been scientifically tested.
- **Authority:** A person with experience and power, who is able to influence the opinions and behavior of other.
- **Bias:** Action or factors other than those investigations that distorts the findings away from truth or expected.
- **Bibliography:** List of publications for a specific topic or specific area.
- **Canonical correlation:** Extension of multiple regressions with more than one dependent variable.
- **Case study:** Intensive and in-depth investigation of a single unit of study.
- **Causality:** Relationship that includes three conditions:
  1. There must be strong correlation between the proposed cause and effect.
  2. The proposed cause must precede the effect in time.
  3. The cause must be present whenever the effect occurs.
- **Cell:** Insertion between the row and column in a table where a specific numerical value is inserted.
- **Code:** Symbol or observation used to clarify words or phrases in qualitative data.
- **Cluster random sampling:** A probability sampling procedure that progress in stages from larger sampling unit to smaller sampling units. It is also called multistage sampling.
- **Cohort:** A group of persons who share a common characteristic such as age, occupation, or area of residence or samples in time dimensional studies within the field or epidemiology.
- **Conclusion:** Synthesis and clarifications of the meaning of study findings.
- **Control group:** The group of elements or subject in which the experimental treatment is not introduced.
- **Conceptual frame work:** Discussion of the relationship of concepts that underline the study problems and support the rational for conducting the study.
- **Confidentiality:** This refers to the assurance given by researchers that data collected from participants will not be revealed to others who are not connected with the study.
- **Correlation:** The statistical association between two or more variables.
- **Data:** Units of information. Singular of data is called datum.
- **Debrief:** To provide subjects of the study with information about the study after the study has been concluded.
- **Demographic variable:** A characteristic or attribute of a study subject such as age, gender, family income, marital status, etc.
- **Dependent variable:** The variable that changes as the independent variable is manipulated by the researcher.

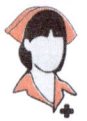

- ❑ **Design:** Blue print for conducting a study, maximizes control over factors that could interfere with the validity of the findings.
- ❑ **Dissertation:** An extensive, usually original research project that is completed by a doctoral student as a part of the requirements for doctoral degree.
- ❑ **Empiricism:** A characteristic of the scientific method in which evidence gathered to generate new knowledge must be rooted in objective reality and must be gathered directly or indirectly through five human senses.
- ❑ **Ethnographic researcher:** Qualitative research mythology for investigating cultures.
- ❑ **Experimental group:** The group in which the experimental treatment is introduced.
- ❑ **Exploratory study:** Study conducted when relatively little is known about the phenomenon.
- ❑ **Factor:** Closely related variables that are grouped together.
- ❑ **Frame work:** Abstract logical structure of meaning such as theory that guides the development of the study.
- ❑ **Frequency:** This involves describing scores in absolute numbers, percentages and proportions.
- ❑ **Grounded theory research:** Inductive research technique based on symbolic interaction theory.
- ❑ **Heterogeneous sample:** A sample in which subjects have a broad range of values being studied, which increases the representativeness of the sample and the ability to generalize from the accessible population to the target population.
- ❑ **Hypothesis:** Formal statement of the expected relationship between two or more variables in a specified population.
- ❑ **Independent groups:** Study groups chosen so that the selection of one subject is unrelated to the selection of other subjects.
- ❑ **Informed consent:** Agreement by a prospective subject to participate voluntarily in a study after he or she has assimilated essential information about the study.
- ❑ **Interview:** Structural or unstructural oral communication between the researcher and the subject during which information is obtained.
- ❑ **Intuition:** Insight or understanding of a situation an event as a whole that usually cannot be logically explained.
- ❑ **Justice, principle:** Ethical principle stating that human subjects should be treated fairly.
- ❑ **Key words:** Major concepts or variables of a research problem or topic that are used to begin a search of a database.
- ❑ **Knowledge:** Information that is acquired in a variety of ways is expected to be an accurate reflection of reality and is incorporated and used to direct a person's action.
- ❑ **Limitations:** Theoretical and methodological restrictions in study that may decrease the generalizability of the findings.
- ❑ **Literature review:** Summary of theoretical and empirical sources to generate a picture of what is known and not known about a particular problem.
- ❑ **Manipulation:** Moving around or controlling a specific attribute of, as in manipulation of a treatment.
- ❑ **Mentor:** Person who provides information, advice and emotional support to a protégé.
- ❑ **Monographs:** Sources that are written once, such as books, booklet of conference proceedings or pamphlets, and may be updated with new addition.

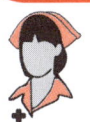

- **Nonprobability sampling:** In which not every element of the population has an opportunity for selection.
- **Null hypothesis:** Hypothesis stating as no relationship exist between the variables being studied.
- **Observation:** Watching and noting action and reactions.
- **Operational definition:** The process of communicating precisely the meaning of concepts and the ways in which they can be observed and recorded.
- **Population:** The total group of individual people or things meeting the designated criteria of interest to the researcher. Typically shown as 'N' or the units from which the data are collected.
- **Primary source:** First-hand information obtained from original material or hearsay information.
- **Periodicals:** Literature sources such as journals that are published one time and are numbered sequentially for the years published.
- **Pilot study:** Smaller version of proposed study or a small-scale version of the actual study conducted with the purpose of testing and potentially refining the research plan.
- **Process:** Purpose, series of actions and goal.
- **Pretest:** The process of testing the effectiveness of a measuring instrument in gathering appropriate data.
- **Qualitative data:** Data characterized by words rather than numbers.
- **Quantitative data:** Data characterized by numbers.
- **Questionnaire:** Printed self-report from designed to elicit information that can be responses of the subject.
- **Range:** This refers to the process of repeating the same study in the same or similar settings using the same method with the same or equivalent sample.
- **Random sampling:** Selection of subjects based on chance alone.
- **Reliability:**
  - In quantitative research, the stability of a measuring instrument over time.
  - In qualitative research, the measure of the extent to which random variation may have influenced stability and consistency of results.
- **Research design:** A plan of how, when and where data are to be collected and analyzed.
- **Research process:** A guide for deriving systematic information concerning the phenomena of research to the researcher.
- **Reliability:** Extent to which an instrument consistently measures a concept.
- **Review of literature:** Summary of current theoretical and empirical sources to generate a picture of what is known and not known about a particular problem.
- **Sample:** A smaller part of the population selected in such a way that the individuals in the sample represent the characteristics of the population. Process of selecting the sample from population is called sampling.
- **Story:** Time bound event shared orally with others.
- **Subjects:** Individuals participating in study.
- **Scale:** Self-report form of measurement composed of several items through to measure the construct being studied.
- **Survey research:** The collection of data directly from the study subjects.

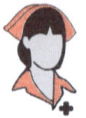

- ❑ **Theoretical definition:** Definition of a variable of interrelated theories being tested in order to support the rational for conducting the study.
- ❑ **Thesis:** Research project completed by a student as a part of the requirement for a master degree.
- ❑ **Triangulation:**
  - The use of both qualitative and quantitative methods in the same research study
  - In quantitative studies, the use of three or more techniques to collect data
- ❑ **Unobtrusive measure:** The researcher decides what needs to be measured and then determines how to measure it without direct intervention.
- ❑ **Utilization:** Used knowledge generated through research to guide nursing practice.
- ❑ **Variance:** Measure of dispersion.
- ❑ **Variable:** An attribute or characteristic that can have more than one value.
- ❑ **Z-score:** Standardized score of the normal curve that is equivalent to the standard deviation of the normal curve.

REVIEW OF LITERATURE

Review of literature is one of the most important steps in research process. The main purpose of the literature review is to convey to the readers about the work already done and the knowledge and ideas that has been already established on particular topic of research. No doubt it is laborious task but essential for the success of research project.

According of ANA (2000), "A literature review is a body of text that aims to review the critical points of knowledge on a particular topic of research."

Importance and Objectives

Literature review is a handy guide to a particular topic which can fulfill the following objectives:
- ❑ Identification of research problem and development of research questions
- ❑ Generation of useful research questions or projects for the discipline
- ❑ Orientation to what is known and not known about topic
- ❑ Determination of any gap or inconsistencies in a body of knowledge
- ❑ Discovery of unanswered questions about subjects, concepts, or problems
- ❑ Identification of relevant theoretical or conceptual framework for research problems
- ❑ Development of hypothesis to be tested in a research study
- ❑ Helps in planning the methodology of the present research study
- ❑ It also helps in development of research instruments
- ❑ Assistance in interpreting study findings and in developing implications and recommendations.

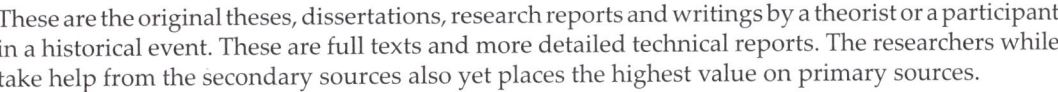

Sources

Primary Sources

These are the original theses, dissertations, research reports and writings by a theorist or a participant in a historical event. These are full texts and more detailed technical reports. The researchers while take help from the secondary sources also yet places the highest value on primary sources.

Secondary Sources

These are the review already done and published by other researches or reviewers on a particular subject or sector of knowledge. These sources are useful because, they provide overview of research developments on a subject and enable the researcher to compile a list of primary sources.

The resources from where the literature review can be get are as follows:
- Electronic sources
- Books
- Journals
- Conference papers
- Thesis
- Encyclopedia and dictionary
- Research reports
- Magazines and newspapers

Steps in a Review of Literature

- Analysis of the problem statement in terms of concepts and variables involved
- Study secondary sources to obtain an overview of the problem for its formulation
- Select relevant indexes
- Select key words from the problem statement and get in touch with the retrieval systems
- Search the indexes manually or through a computer to prepare a bibliography
- Study the primary sources and take notes on cards
- Arrange and organize the note cards according to ideas concepts, design, etc.
- Arrive at general conclusions of the review and identification of gaps in knowledge.

Types of Literature Review

- The word "empirical" is defined as knowledge derived from research. Other types of published information, such as descriptions of clinical situations, educational literature and position papers, are examined by the researcher in the process of reviewing the literature but are rarely cited in a research publication because of their subjectivity.
- Published studies, usually in journals or books, and unpublished studies, such as master's thesis and dissertations.

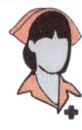

Points to be Considered for Literature Review

Here are some points which should be considered while doing the literature review:

- ❑ Be specific and be succinct
- ❑ Be selective
- ❑ Focus of current topics
- ❑ Ensure evidence for claims
- ❑ Focus on sources of evidences
- ❑ Account of contrary evidences
- ❑ Reference citation
- ❑ Organization of literature review
- ❑ Referring original source
- ❑ Avoid abbreviations
- ❑ Simple and accurate sentence structure.

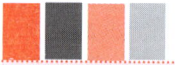 **ASSESS YOURSELF**

1. Define research process.
2. What are the steps to be followed for writing a problem statement?
3. What are the steps of qualitative research process?
4. What are the characteristics of the research objectives?

Research Approaches/ Research Design

6

Learning Objectives

To describe the research approaches.

To discuss the research design.

Key Terms

- **Research design:** A blue print to conduct a study.
- **Control:** The process of holding constant confounding influences on dependent variables under study.
- **Manipulation**: An intervention introduced by the researcher in an experimental study to assess its impact on the dependent variable.

Research design and research approaches terms are used interchangeably. The research design is the plan, structure and strategy of investigations of answering the research questions. It is the overall plan or blue print the researchers select to carry out their study.

There are two main purposes of the research design/approach.

1. To provide answers to research questions.
2. To control variance.

TYPES OF RESEARCH DESIGN

A good research design includes several elements:

- ❑ Description of subject 'who'
- ❑ Observation of variable 'what'
- ❑ Measures of time 'when'
- ❑ Selection of setting 'where'
- ❑ Role of investigator 'how'

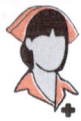

SELECTING A RESEARCH DESIGN

While seeking research design the researcher has to weight many considerations. The factors influence on the research design are given below:

- ❑ Level of knowledge
- ❑ Nature of the phenomena
- ❑ Nature of the purpose
- ❑ Ethical consideration
- ❑ Feasibility
- ❑ Availability of subjects
- ❑ Availability of facility and equipment
- ❑ Validity of data
- ❑ Precision
- ❑ Researcher's experiment
- ❑ Cost
- ❑ Control

These all factors help to select a research design.

TYPES OF RESEARCH APPROACH (FLOW CHART 1)

There are two types of research approaches. They are:

Flow chart 1: Types of research approach

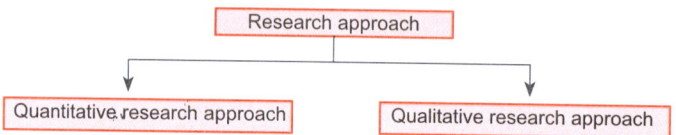

Quantitative Research Approach (Design)

The quantitative research involves a formal, objective systematic process that uses numerical data and statistical procedures to describe or assess relationship between and among variable.

The main types of quantitative research approaches are:

- ❑ **Experimental research**
    - ▪ True experimental
        - o Pre-test/post-test control group design
        - o Solomon four group design
        - o Two group random sample design
        - o Matching sample design
        - o Factorial design
    - ▪ Quasi experimental
        - o One group pre-test/post-test design
        - o Nonrandomized control group design

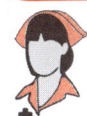

- o Counter balanced design
- o Time series design
- o Control group design
- o Control group series design

The term experiment is scientific investigation in which observations are made and data are collected according to a set of well-defined criteria.

The experimental design is by the following properties:

- ❑ Manipulation
- ❑ Control
- ❑ Randomization
- ❑ Nonexperimental quantitative design:
  - ▪ Co-relational design
  - ▪ Descriptive design
  - ▪ Time perspective design
  - ▪ Retrospective design
  - ▪ Prospective design
  - ▪ Design that use existing data
  - ▪ Focus group research
  - ▪ Content analysis

Qualitative Research Approach

Qualitative research relies less on numbers and measurements and more on observations and interpersonal. Communication that provide a view of the subject's experiences without limiting questions or responses.

The types of qualitative research are:

- ❑ Phenomenological
- ❑ Grounded theory
- ❑ Historical
- ❑ Action research

Advantages and Disadvantages of Qualitative and Quantitative Research Designs

Qualitative research is a systematic, interactive, subjective approach used to describe life experience and give them meaning whereas quantitative research is formal, objective and systematic process to describe, test relationships and examine cause and effects interaction among variables.

Quantitative research is based on the measurement of quantity or amount and it is applicable to phenomena that can be exposed in terms of quantity. Qualitative research on the other hand is concerned with qualitative phenomena, relating to an involving quality or kind.

These two qualitative and quantitative approaches have emerged in recent years to develop nursing knowledge.

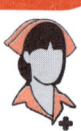

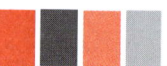 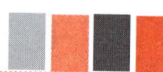

ASSESS YOURSELF

1. Define research design.
2. Enlist factors which influence the research design.
3. What are the types of research approach?
4. Give details about the quantitative research approach/design.

Data Collection Process

7

Learning Objectives

- Explain the sampling process.
- Describe the methods of data collection.

Key Terms

- **Population:** The entire set of individual having some common characters.
- **Sample:** A subset of population selected to participate in study.
- **Data:** The piece of information obtained in study.
- **Validity:** Refers to the degree to which an instrument measures, what it is supposed to be measured.
- **Scales:** A set of symbols or numerals constructed so that these can be assigned by to rule to characteristics of individuals to whom scale is applied.

Data means information that is systematically collected during the course of study. It is an observable and measurable fact. It provides information about the phenomenon under study.

Mainly two types of the data are collected in research: Primary data and Secondary data. Variety of data collection methods are used in nursing research studies such as interview, questionnaires, observation, biophysical measurements, psychological measurement scales, record analysis, etc.

SOURCES OF DATA COLLECTION

Mainly two broad categories are the sources for data collection. These are:

1. **Primary source:** Data that is obtained directly from an individual research unit, objects, program or institution is called primary source. Primary sources provide the first hand information. The recent census is an example of the primary data. It may be collected through interviews, questionnaires, observation, biochemical measurements and psychological measurement scale.

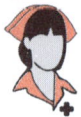

2. **Secondary sources:** Data that is obtained from outside source is called secondary data. This is of two types:
   (i) Internal sources like private documents (Biographies, diaries, letters, memories).
   (ii) External sources like public documents for example, published records and unpublished records (journals, newspaper, government reports, mass communication, unpublished thesis, official or patient records, etc. and internet).

METHODS AND TOOLS OF DATA COLLECTION

Data collection means identification of subjects and the precise, systematic gathering of information (data) relevant to the research purpose or the specific objectives, questions or hypothesis of the study.

The main methods and techniques of data collection are interview, questioning (self-report), observation, biophysiological methods and other methods.

Different tools are used to collect the data from different methods, for example, for the observation method the tools for data collection are rating scales, check lists, anecdotes, videotapes, films and close circuit T.V.

Methods of Data Collection (Flow Chart 1)

Flow chart 1: Techniques of data collections

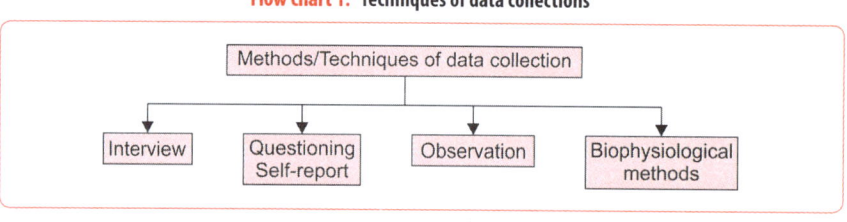

Tools of Data Collection

Tools	Methods/Techniques of data collection
• Interview schedule • Opinionnaire	Interview
• Questionnaire • Likert scale and Semantic differential scale • Visual analogue scale	Questioning (Self-report)
• Rating scale • Checklist • Anecdotes • Videotape films • CCTVs	Observation
• *In vivo* biophysiological measurements • *In vitro* biophysiological measurements	Biophysiological measurements

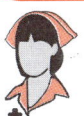

Selection of the Methods of Data Collection

Appropriate and complete answer of research questions largely depends upon the selection of appropriate method of data collection. Factors influencing data collection are as follows:

- ❑ The nature of phenomenon under study
- ❑ Type of research subjects
- ❑ The type of research study
- ❑ The purpose of research study
- ❑ Size of the study sample
- ❑ Distribution of the target population
- ❑ Time frame of the study
- ❑ Literacy level of the subjects
- ❑ Availability of resources and man power
- ❑ Research knowledge level and competence.

INTERVIEW METHOD

Interview comes under the primary data collection. It is a method in which one person (interviewer) asks the questions from another person (respondent); which is conducted either face to face or telephonically. It is the only suitable method for gathering the data from the illiterate and less educated respondents. Once rapport is established, even confidential information can be obtained.

Aims of Interview

The major aims of interview are:

- ❑ To secure information through face to face association and thereby gain the portrait of the entire personality, broad enough to encompass the social and psychological background.
- ❑ To form a hypothesis.
- ❑ To collect personal data for quantitative purpose.
- ❑ To collect data from persons who are secondary sources of information.

Kinds of Interview

Social scientists have described four kinds of interview:

1. **Direct or structured interview:** A schedule containing a set of predetermined questions is prepared. The researcher has to get the answers of these questions only even without adding, deleting or even altering the language.
2. **Nondirective or unstructured interview:** No predetermined questions are asked. The researcher collects information by free discussion. The subject is asked to narrate in his own words his experiences, opinions or reactions under research.
3. **Focused interview:** This type of interview is generally used to study the social and psychological effects of mass communication.
4. **Repetitive interview:** It is used when it is desired to note the gradual influence of some social or psychological process.

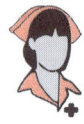

Technique of Interview

Conducting an interview is both an art and science. Sociologist have described the following steps for conducting an interview:

- ❑ Establishing contacts
- ❑ Starting an interview
- ❑ Securing rapport
- ❑ Recall
- ❑ Probe questions
- ❑ Encouragement
- ❑ Guiding the interview
- ❑ Recording
- ❑ Closing the interview
- ❑ Report

Planning for the interview time, place, questions, mode of recording, etc. should be done. Seeking to interviewee's permission or approval and fixing up time, etc. for the interview should be done. To decrease the anxiety and explaining the purpose of interview a good rapport should be established. Then the interview according to need should be done. Recording of the interview should be done as required like mechanically, electronically, etc. In the end of the interview the termination should be done with a word of thanks. After that interpretation and analysis of interview should be done.

Advantages

- ❑ As interview is a personal contact method. More information in depth can be obtained.
- ❑ Ambiguous or confusing questions can be reconstruct as there is greater flexibility in this method, especially in the case of unstructured interviews.
- ❑ Interview permits greater control over the samples.
- ❑ Samples can be controlled more effectively as there arises no difficulty of the missing returns; non-response generally remains very low.
- ❑ Higher proportions of responses are obtained from potential respondents.
- ❑ It is highly useful for working with the illiterate, the young children and mental defective respondents.
- ❑ It is flexible and adaptable in various situations.
- ❑ It can be used as the main tool of research.

Disadvantages

- ❑ An individual interview is very much time consuming.
- ❑ Client and researcher bias chances are more.
- ❑ It is difficult to record, analyze and interpret.
- ❑ It is a costly affair.
- ❑ Different interviewers may understand and translate interviews in different ways.
- ❑ The respondent may hide few things due to shyness and hesitation.
- ❑ Interview cannot be used for all types of research problem.

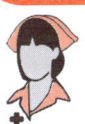

OBSERVATION METHOD

Observation is a data collection method which is used by the researcher. The investigator collects the requisite information personally through observation. Observation is a way of gathering the data by watching behavior, events or noting physical characteristics in their natural setting. This type of data collection is particularly well suited to nursing research.

Observations can be overt (everyone knows they are being observed) and covert (they do not know that they are being observed and the observer is concealed).

Observation can also be either direct or indirect. Direct observation is when you watch interactions, processes and behavior as they occur. Indirect observations are when you watch the results of interaction, processes, or behavior.

Definition

Observation is a technique for collecting all the data or acquiring information through occurrences that can be observed through senses with or without mechanical devices. It is two-part process to collect data for study that includes an observer (someone who is observing) and the observed.

Types

- **Structured observation:** In this method, a structured or semi-structured tool is prepared in advance to observe the phenomenon under study. The researcher has to observe only specific attributes or behaviors in accordance with preplanned structured or semi-structured instruments and guidelines. It is generally carried out by using following tools:
  - Checklist
  - Rating scale
  - Category system
- **Unstructured observation:** It is used in qualitative studies. Observation is made with unstructured tools and used for complete and non-specific observation of phenomenon, which is well known by the researcher. The tools may be:
  - Log and field notes: Log notes are the notes which are recorded in log books
  - Anecdotes
  - Field dairy
  - Notes
  - Photographs, tap recording
  - Video recording
- **Participant observation:** The observer becomes the part of the group or activity which he wants to observe. The persons observed are generally not aware of his presence as an observer. He becomes the accepted member of the group. Unstructured tools are used to collect the data.
- **Nonparticipant observation:** This is generally done by the observation by keeping out of the group or the activity, i.e. the observer is not a participant in the setting but nearly viewing the situation. This method is mostly used by the psychologists for the children and animals.

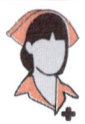

Steps in Developing an Observation Schedule

- **Select the focus:** Selecting the aspect of the behavior to be observed a systematic and categories of behavior should be selected which is to be observed. As one person cannot record everything, we notice.

- **Training observer:** It is critical that the observer is well trained in your data collection process to ensure high quality and consistent data. The level of training will be based on the complexity of the data collection and the individual capabilities of observe. The difficulties can be resolved through discussions and the practice sessions.

- **Recording:** In order to have adequate account of what was observed during observation same procedure recording should be followed, either during the observation or soon after the observation is completed. This requires advance planning.

- **Testing observation schedule:** Systematic examination of the observation schedule should be done to ascertain the adequacy of content being put to measure:
  - The observations under taken are consistent with the study's specific objectives
  - There is standardized and systematic plan for the observation and the recording of data
  - All of the observations are checked and controlled
  - The observations are related to the scientific and theories.

  Thus, scientific observation requires preplanning systematic recording controlling the observation and relationship to scientific theory.

- **Tools for observation:** As scientific observation needs to be recorded with preplanning. Certain tools are required. The main tools are as follows:
  - **Anecdotes:** A typically selected specific kind of events and behaviors are taken before hand and focus is made on behavior of particular interest. The observer has to record the observations objectively and accurately.
  - **Rating scale:** Rating scale refers to a scale with a set of opinion, which describes varying degree of the dimensions of an attitude being observed. Rating scales are value judgments about attributes of one person to another person. These scales are most commonly used tools to carry out structural observations.

    Rating scales have the following types:
    - Graphic rating scale
    - Descriptive rating scale
    - Numerical rating scale
    - Comparative rating scale

  The rating scale should be used accurately as there are chances of subjective evaluation, thus scale may become unscientific and unreliable.

- **Check list:** It is one of the most commonly used instruments for performance evaluation. It is a simple instrument consisting prepared list of expected items of performance or attributes, which are checked by a researcher for their presence or absence. The observer should be trained how to observe, what to observe, and how to record the observed behavior. Checklist is very useful in evaluating procedural works and learning activities. The main disadvantage of checklist is, it does not indicate quality of the performance so only a limited components or performance parameter may be assessed.

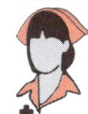

Advantages of Observation

❑ Where and when an event or activity is occurring collection of data can be done
❑ Provide depth and variety of information
❑ Does not rely on people's willingness or ability to provide information
❑ It is an important technique for studying human behavior especially where interventions are used
❑ It is open to use of recording devices such as tape recorder and the cameras
❑ One can make use of assistants to carry out observations.

Disadvantages of Observation

❑ Just susceptible to observer bias.
❑ Lack of consent to being observed cannot be ignored for the ethical reasons.
❑ Time and duration of the event cannot be predicted as observer has to wait for an event to be happen.
❑ Susceptible to the 'Hawthorne effect', that is, people usually perform better when they knew they are being observed, although indirect observation may decrease this problem.
❑ Observed events are subjected to researcher's cultural background and personal interpretation.
❑ Uses of recording devices are expensive.
❑ Assistant observer if used than extensive training for him/her is must.

QUESTIONNAIRE

In the observation method, it may be difficult to produce accurate data due to physical difficulties and perception which can lead to the errors. Because of these limitations *questionnaire method* is more widely used for the data collection. In this method the researcher prepares a sequence of relevant questions which he/she wants to ask about his sample. Then the clients can respond it and researcher can record the responses. Questionnaire method can be applied through personal interview, by mail or telephonically.

The questionnaire may have three main aspects:

1. The general form of questionnaire which depends upon the type of data the researcher wants. Mainly it is of two types they are *structured questionnaire* and *unstructured questionnaire.*
    (i) **Structured questionnaire:** As name indicates the questions and answers are specified and the respondents has to give only very limited comments. Only very specific information can be sort out from such questionnaire.
    (ii) **Unstructured questionnaire:** It is very useful for the depth interviews or the interviews where we can probe or see the general response of the sample. These are open ended type questions and the samples have full liberty to comment on the questions.

    The main drawback of unstructured questionnaire is that it cannot be mailed as mail questionnaire method of data collection.

2. **The question sequence:** Proper sequence of the questions keep the interest of the respondent intact. The introductory questions should be as short and simple as possible. The covering letter or introductory letter should highlight the purpose of study and assure the respondent that responses will be kept confidential. It should be brief.

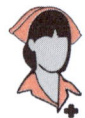

Once the rapport with the respondent is established then the questions should be started from easy to complex form. Personal questions like wealth or character should be avoided in the beginning. The questionnaire should be pretested before mailing or administration.

3. **The question wording:** The words can win the world or the words can be more sharper than sword. The wording of the questions should be chosen with great care and control. The framing of question wording should be strictly according to the study and should be impartial. Unwanted data or phases should be avoided. In general, the question should be as follows:

- They can be easily understood by respondent.
- They should be simple and convey only one thought at a time.
- They should be concrete and conform to respondent's way of thinking.
- Words with ambiguous meaning should be avoided.

Steps in the Construction of a Questionnaire

- ❏ The questionnaire must be developed exactly in accordance with study objectives
- ❏ Typed questions should be decided
- ❏ Use statement which can be interpreted in same way by all subjects
- ❏ Questions should flow from general to more specific and from least to most sensitive
- ❏ Questionnaire should be brief
- ❏ Avoid asking double barreled questions which contain two district ideas or concepts
- ❏ Avoid negative questions or statements
- ❏ Use correct spelling, grammar and punctuation.
- ❏ Every questionnaire should have an appropriate ending.

Types of Questions

Mainly questions which are used in questionnaire method are of three types:
1. Open format questions.
2. Closed ended questions.
3. Pictorial form questions.

Open Format Questions

Open ended questions provide opportunity to the respondents to express their opinions and answers in their own way. There is no predetermined set of responses. They provide true, insightful and unexpected suggestions.

Advantages

- ❏ The open form questionnaire is good for depth studies
- ❏ Freedom to the respondents to answer the questions without any restriction
- ❏ Easy to construct.

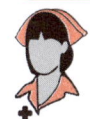

Disadvantages

- Analysis is difficult and time consuming
- It is less efficient in the sense respondents take more time
- The respondent may nerve be aware of all the possible answers.

Closed Ended Questions

These questions offer respondents a number of alternative replies, from which the subjects must choose the one that most likely matches the appropriate answer.

Close ended questions could be of following subtypes:

- Dichotomous questions
- Multiple choice questions
- Cafeteria questions
- Rank order questions
- Contingency questions
- Rating questions
- Likert questions
- Matrix questions

Advantages

- Close end questions facilitate easy statistical calculation of data
- It provides easy preliminary analysis
- Less time consuming for the respondents
- It is easy to fill out
- Relatively objective, and fairly more convenient for tabulation and analysis.

Disadvantages

- It is difficult to construct
- This type of questions are superficial
- This may involve selecting from a limited choice or rating, which does not satisfy the respondent.

Pictorial form Questions

Pictorial questionnaires contain drawing photographs or other such material instead of written statements. Instructions and directions can be given orally. This is very useful for the illiterate, young children and persons not knowing a specific language.

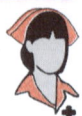

Advantages

- Questionnaire are cost effective
- They are easy to analyze
- Simple, quick and inexpensive method of obtaining data
- Questionnaires are used for large sample size
- They reduce bias as interview method.

Disadvantages

- Low response rate
- Unable to probe a topic in depth
- Respondent may omit any item without giving any explanation
- Printing may be costly
- There are chances of misinterpretation
- If respondent is promised anonymity, it is impossible to know who returned the questionnaire in case follow-up is needed.

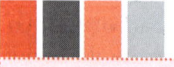 **ASSESS YOURSELF**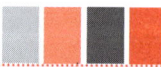

1. Define sources of data collection.
2. Enlist the factors influencing the selection of the methods of data collections.
3. Write advantages and disadvantages of interview method of data collection.
4. Write the steps to contract a questionnaire.

Analysis of Data

8

Learning Objectives

- To analyze the data.
- To interpret the data.
- To summarize the research data.

Key Terms

- **Analysis:** Computation, finding relation along the data available.
- **Tabulation:** Recording of the classified material in accurate mathematical terms with the help of rows and columns.

COMPILATION

Compilation is a process, which includes gathering together all the collected data in a manner, that is process of analysis can be initiated. While compiling the data, care is to be taken to arrange all data in order so that editing and coding process can be implemented with ease.

The analysis of data is a process which requires creativity, conceptual sensitivity, and sheer hard work. The main purpose of data analysis is to organize, provide structure and elicit meaning from the data.

PRESENTATION OF STATISTICAL DATA

Data obtained by the investigator is irregularly documented and is unorganized known as the raw data. This raw data should be organized for the analysis in a specific sequence and should be presented in such a way as to make it easily understandable.

There are mainly three forms of representing the data:

1. Tabular form
2. Graphic form
3. Diagrammatic form

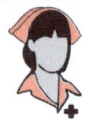

TABULATION OR TABULAR FORM

Tables are the devices to present the statistical data in frequently arranged form. These tables help to give maximum information in easily understood way. The tables can be simple or complex depends upon the number of measurements. Following principles and points should be kept in mind while constructing a table:

Principles for Designing Tables

- ❑ Tables should be numbered, e.g. Table 1, Table 2, etc.
- ❑ A brief, self-explanatory title should be given to every table
- ❑ Concise and clear headings should be given to columns and rows
- ❑ The data must be presented according to size or importance, chronologically, alphabetically or geographically
- ❑ If percentage or average are to be compared they should be placed as close as possible
- ❑ No table should be too large
- ❑ Vertical arrangements are considered better than horizontal arrangements by most of the people, because it is easy to scan the data from top to bottom than from left to right.
- ❑ Foot notes may be given, where necessary, providing notes.

Manual Tabulation

The process of tabulation is simple and does not require any technical knowledge or skill.

Computerized Tabulation

Computerized tabulation is very easy with the help of computer software packages. A set of integrated programs suitable for analysis of data is there. These packages contains programs for a wide range of operations and analysis such as handling missing data, recording, variable information, simple descriptive analysis, cross tabulation, multivariate analysis and non-parametric analysis. Tabulating machines and other mechanical devices to tabulating are coming into use which are very quick and precise.

Tabulations are devices for presenting data from a mass of statistical data. Some examples of the both types (Simple and complex) in which vital statistics are presenting. They are as under:

Simple Table

In this table only one type of data or characteristics are presented. They are also called single characteristic table, e.g. marks obtained in Math test

Roll No.	Marks obtained out of 50
01	40
02	45
03	48

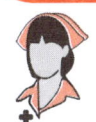

Frequency Distribution Table or Complex Table

In a complex or frequency distribution table, the data is first split up into convenient groups (class intervals) and the number of items (frequency) which occur in each group is shown in adjacent column.

Example: The following figures are the ages of patients admitted to a hospital with poliomyelitis. Construct a frequency distribution table.

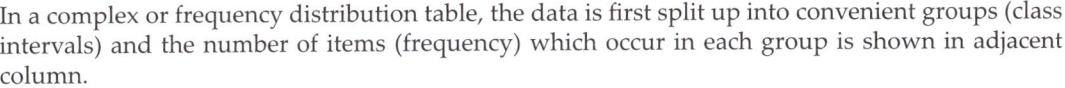

8, 24, 18, 5, 6, 12, 4, 3, 3, 2, 3, 23, 9, 18, 16, 1, 2, 3, 5, 11,
13, 15, 9, 11, 11, 7, 10, 6, 9, 5, 16, 20, 4, 3, 3, 3, 10, 3, 2, 1,
6, 9, 3, 7, 14, 8, 1, 4, 6, 4, 15, 22, 2, 1, 4, 7, 1, 12, 3, 23,
4, 19, 6, 2, 2, 4, 14, 2, 2, 21, 3, 2, 9, 3, 2, 1, 7, 19

The given data can be conveniently analyzed as shown below:

Age group	Tally	Frequency
0–4	ⅢⅢ ⅢⅢ ⅢⅢ ⅢⅢ ⅢⅢ ⅢⅢ ⅢⅢ	35
5–9	ⅢⅢ ⅢⅢ ⅢⅢ III	18
10–14	ⅢⅢ ⅢⅢ I	11
15–19	ⅢⅢ III	8
20–24	ⅢⅢ I	6

The data, analyzed above, is prepared in the form of a frequency table as shown below:

Age	No. of patients
0–4	35
5–9	18
10–14	11
15–19	8
20–24	6

In the above example, the age is split into group of five. These are known as **class intervals**. The number of observation in each group is called frequency. In constructing frequency distribution table we should able to know:

- ❑ Into how many groups the date should be split?
- ❑ What class intervals should be chosen?

As a practical rule, it might be stated that when there is large data, a maximum of 20 groups, and when there is not much data, a minimum of 5 groups, could be conveniently taken. As far as possible, the class intervals should be equal, so that observations could be compared.

Merits of Tabulation

The advantages of presenting statistical data in tabular form are so obvious as to make extended comment unnecessary.

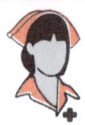

It might, however, to point out that:

- Statistical tables conserve space and reduce explanatory and descriptive statements to a minimum
- The visualization of relations and the process of comparison is greatly facilitated by tables
- Tabulated data can be more easily remembered than data which are not tabulated
- A tabular arrangement facilitates the summation of items and the detection of errors and omissions
- Statistical totals provide a basis for computations. Tables are devices for presenting data simply from masses of statistical data
- It saves space
- Lengthy explanatory and descriptive statements reduced in length with self-explanation
- It facilitates to detection and omission of errors
- Further statistical computation becomes easier
- The tables show the range, and the shape of distribution
- The table should be made as logical, clear, accurate and simple as possible.

CHARTS AND DIAGRAMS

Some general rules for graphic representation:

- Each chart or diagram should have a title which should be written above the contents
- The title should have following qualities:
  - Clear
  - Concise
  - Simple
  - Describe nature of data presented.
- Numerical data should also be presented in table form along chart or diagram
- Horizontal lines are for independent variables whereas the vertical lines measured variables
- Each curve, line, bar should be properly labeled
- If more than one structures are present these should be differentiated from one another either by colors or designs
- Zero point should always represented in center, from where the scale intervals can be kept equal
- Too many graphic forms should be avoided
- Graphic form should be made before the textual discussion
- This representation of charts and diagrams, no doubt is simple but it can hide some original details. So for the deep studies the original data should also be seen.

BAR CHART

Bar charts or Bar diagrams consists of equally spaced vertical rectangular bar of equal width placed on common horizontal base. The heights of the rectangles are proportional to the frequencies. The vertical bars substitute the straight lines. Bar charts/Diagrams are easy to prepare and understand.

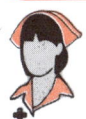

These charts enable values to be compared visually. There are three types of Bar charts.

- Simple Bar chart
- Multiple Bar chart
- Divided or Component Bar chart

Simple Bar Chart

This type of bar chart is used to compare two or more items related to a variable. Bars may be vertical or horizontal as (Figs 1 and 2). The suitable scale should be chosen for the diagram.

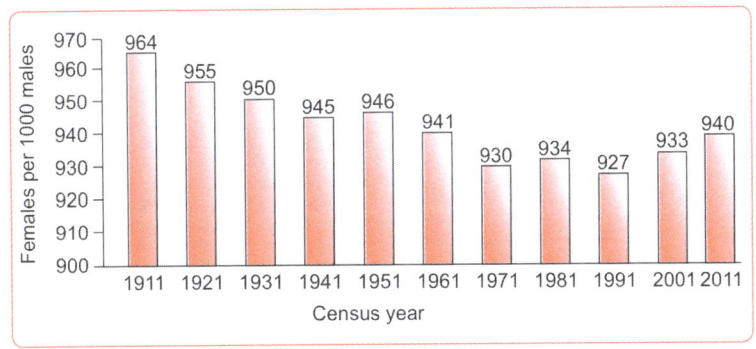

Fig. 1:   India—Sex ratio from 1911–2011

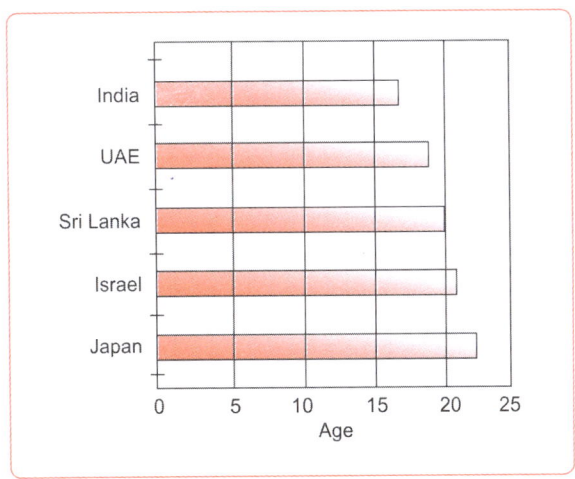

Fig. 2:   Mean age at marriage (females) in some countries

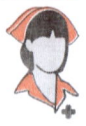

Multiple Bar Chart

A multiple bar diagram (Fig. 3) is used when a number of items are to be compared in respect of two, three or more values. This can be distinguished by different colors or patterns for each character.

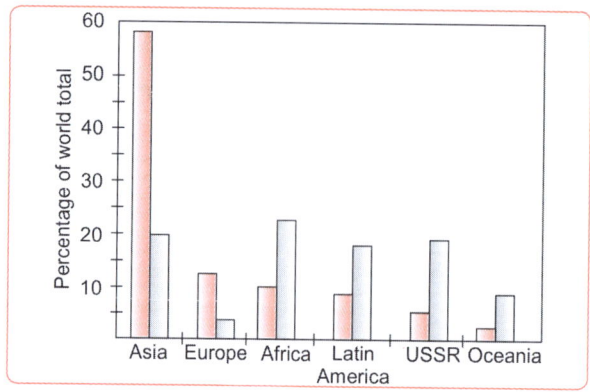

Fig. 3: Population and land area by region

Component Bar Chart

A divided or component bar diagram can be formed by dividing a single bar represents the aggregate value, whereas the component parts represent the component values of the aggregate value (Fig. 4).

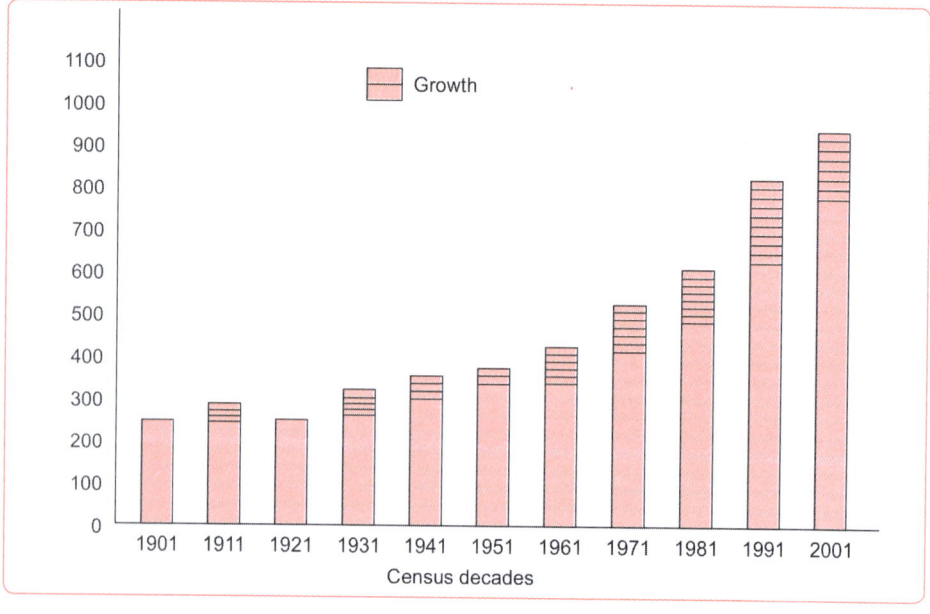

Fig. 4: India: Growth of population 1901 to 2001

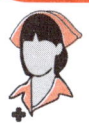

HISTOGRAM

A histogram is a series of rectangles having areas that is in the same proportion as the frequencies of a frequency distribution. Figure 5 shows histogram of the frequency distribution of blood pressure in females 45–65 years.

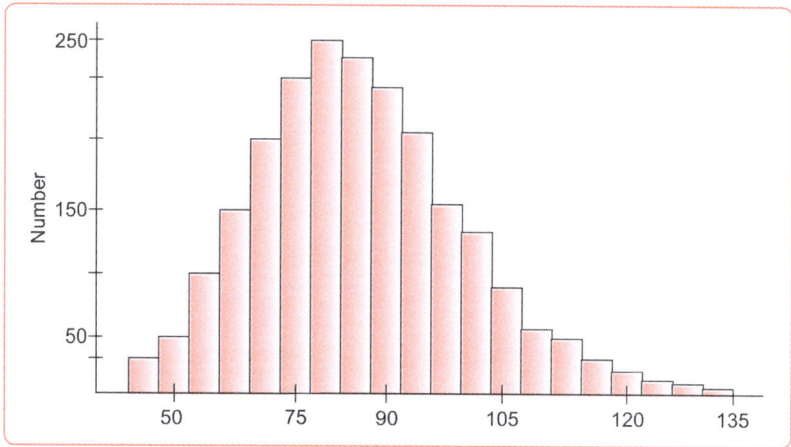

Fig. 5: **Frequency distribution of diastolic blood pressure in females aged 45–65 years**

LINE DIAGRAM

These form the simplest way of diagrammatic representation of data. Discrete variables are plotted against x-axis and frequencies are plotted against y-axis. Figure 6 shows the trend of malaria cases reported throughout the world during 1972 to 1978.

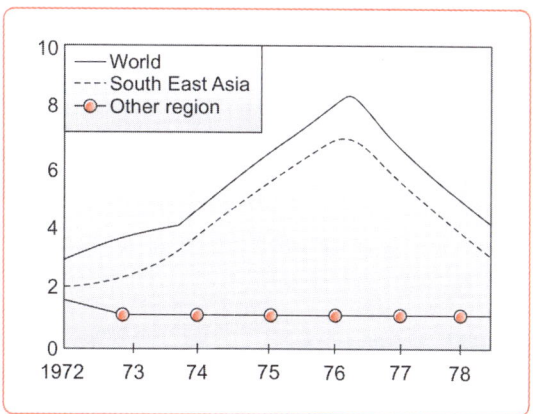

Fig. 6: Malaria cases reported throughout the world during 1972–1978 (excluding African region)

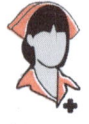

PIE CHART

A pie chart is also known as circular chart or sector chart. It is used for percentage distribution. Different components are represented by means of sectors of the circle (Fig. 7).

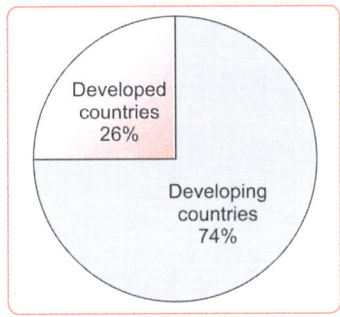

Fig. 7: Pie diagram of world population

PICTOGRAM

It is the popular method of presenting data from the old time. Small pictures or symbols are used to present the data. It is a method to impress the frequency of occurrence of the events to common man. The following rules should be observed in developing the pictogram:

❏ The symbols should be self-explanatory
❏ Each symbol should represent a convenient sum of units
❏ The chart should be made as simple and clear as possible
❏ The chart should give only on overall picture; it should not show minute details
❏ Comparison in terms of one dimension only should be charted. For example, a picture of a doctor to represent the population per physician (Fig. 8).

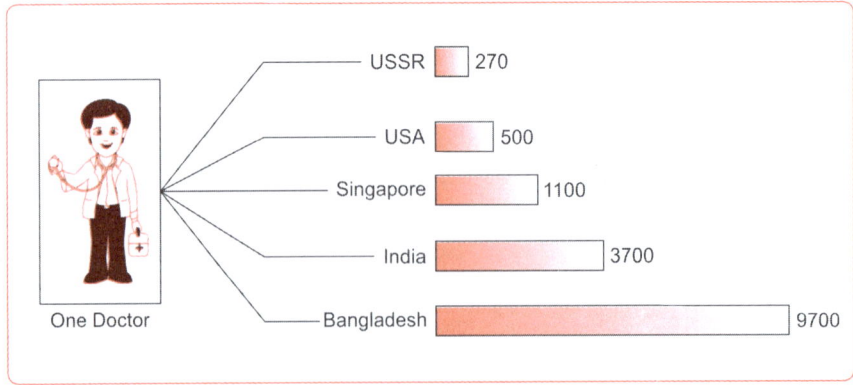

Fig. 8: A pictogram: Population per physician

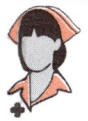

STATISTICAL MAPS

Geographical or administrative area data is presented either as shaded maps or dot maps. The shaded maps are used to present data of varying size. The areas are shaded with the different colors or different intensity of same color which is indicated in the key. For example, Master rotation plan or clinical rotation plans.

SCATTER DIAGRAM

It shows the relationship between two variables. If the dots cluster around a straight line it shows evidence of a linear nature. It there is no such cluster, it is probable that there is no relationship between the variables.

STATISTICAL AVERAGES

The average lies somewhere within the range of data. Because of this, the statistical average is also described as measures of central tendency.

Measures of Central Tendency

When a researcher collects the values of any characteristics, we can see that observation values cluster around a central value. This property of concentration of the value around a central value is known as central tendency. This can be measured by measuring mean, median and mode.

Mean

Mean is the mathematical average. There are mainly three types of mathematical averages or mean. They are:

❑ Arithmetic mean
❑ Geometric mean
❑ Harmonic mean

Mainly mean is the measure of center of set of values. It is denoted by sign Σ or S.

The mean is denoted by $\bar{X}$ (called $\bar{X}$ bar)

For example:

$$\bar{X} = \frac{X_1 + X_2 + X_3 + X_4 - - - - - - - - X_n}{n} = \frac{\Sigma X}{n}$$

where $\bar{X}$ is mean
X_1, X_2 ------ = Different values
n = Number of observations

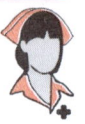

Advantages

It has certainty. Mean can never be biased. Simple to calculate. Easy to understand. It is based on observations.

Disadvantages

- ❑ It cannot be used for small number of classes.
- ❑ It cannot be used for qualitative characters.

Median

The value which divides the whole data into two equal parts is known as median, if the values are arranged in ascending or descending order of magnitude. It is the value of the middle observation.

$$\text{Median} = \frac{\text{Number of observations} + 1}{2} = \left[\frac{n+1}{2}\right]^{th} \text{observations}$$

Diastolic blood pressure
71
75
75
77
79 medium
81
83
84
95

Data arranged in order of magnitude.

Advantages

- ❑ It is useful in case of open ended classes and unequal classes.
- ❑ Extreme values do not affect median.
- ❑ It is the most appropriate average in dealing with qualitative data. The main disadvantage of median is that

Disadvantages

- ❑ For calculation of median it is necessary to arrange the data.
- ❑ It is not capable of further algebraic treatment.
- ❑ Median is not calculated for quantitative data.

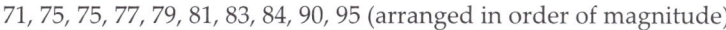
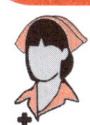

If the values are in even number, i.e. 10 instead of 9 then the medium is worked out by taking average of the two middle values.

For example, if we add one more frequency, i.e. 90 in the above data and make 10 observations instead of 9 then the median will be

71, 75, 75, 77, 79, 81, 83, 84, 90, 95 (arranged in order of magnitude)

$$\text{Median} = \frac{79 + 81}{2} = 80$$

Mode

The mode is the commonly occurring value in the distribution of data. It is the most frequent item of the most fashionable value in the series of observations.

For example: The diastolic blood pressure of 20 individuals is given as following. Find the mode.

85, 75, 81, 79, 71, 95, 75, 77, 75, 90, 71, 75, 79, 95, 75, 77, 84, 75, 81, 75

So the mode is the most frequently occurring figure that is 75.

Advantages

It is easily to understand and not affected by extreme items.

Disadvantages

The exact location is often uncertain and is often not clearly defined. Therefore mode is often not used in medical or biological statistics.

MEASUREMENT OF DISPERSION

The observation deviating from the central value is different in different sets of values of character. In the same distributions, the difference may be less, whereas in others may be more. This property of deviation of the values from the average is called variation or dispersion. The degree of variation is indicated by measure of dispersion. The various measures of the dispersion are:

- ❑ Range
- ❑ Mean or average deviation
- ❑ Standard deviation

Range

The range is by far the simplest measure of dispersion. It is defined as the difference between highest and lowest figures in a given sample.

Range (R) = (H) – (L) where H is the highest figure and L is the lowest figure in the given sample.

Example for range: Calculate the range of the data for the diastolic blood pressure of 10 individuals

83, 75, 81, 79, 71, 90, 75, 95, 77, 95

The range will be R = H – L = R = 95 – 71 = 24

So the range is 24.

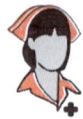

Advantages

❑ It is very simple to understand
❑ Very easy to calculate

Disadvantages

❑ It is not suitable for deep analysis and
❑ Not suitable in the case of extreme values.

Mean Deviation

It is the average of the deviation from the arithmetic mean. It is given by the formula

$$MD = \sum \frac{(x - \bar{x})}{\eta}$$

For example: The diastolic blood pressure of 10 individuals is as follows:

83, 75, 81, 79, 71, 95, 75, 77, 84 and 90

Find the mean deviation.

Diastolic BP X	Arithmetic mean $\bar{X}$	Deviation from the mean $(X - \bar{X})$
83	81	2
75	81	−6
81	81	0
79	81	−2
71	81	−10
95	81	14
75	81	−6
77	81	−4
84	81	3
90	81	9
Total 810		Total = 56
Mean $\frac{810}{10} = 81$		(Ignoring ± sign)

So the mean deviation is $\frac{56}{10} = 5.6$

Standard Deviation

Standard deviation is the most frequently used measure of deviation. In simple terms, it is defined as "Root – mean – square – deviation". It is denoted by a Greek letter sigma (σ) by the initials SD.

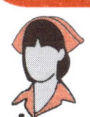

The standard deviation (SD) is calculated from the basic formula:

$$SD = \sqrt{\frac{\Sigma(X-\bar{X})^2}{\eta}}$$

When the sample size is more than 30, the above basic formula may be used without modification. For smaller sample, the formula tends to underestimate the standard deviation and therefore needs correction, which is done by substituting the denomination $(\eta-1)$ for η. The modified formula is as follows:

$$SD = \sqrt{\frac{\Sigma(X-\bar{X})^2}{\eta-1}}$$

The steps involved in calculating the standard deviation are as following:

a. First of all, take the deviation of each value from the arithmetic mean
$(X-\bar{X})$
b. Then square each deviation
$(X-\bar{X})^2$
c. Add up the squared deviation
$\Sigma(X-\bar{X})^2$
d. Divide the result by number of observations η

Then take the square root, which gives the standard deviation

For example: The diagnostic blood pressure of some of the individuals is as follows:

83, 75, 81, 79, 71, 95, 75, 77, 84, 90

Find out the standard deviation.

X	X – X̄	(X – X̄)²
83	2	4
75	–6	36
81	0	–
79	–2	4
71	–10	100
95	14	196
75	6	36
77	4	16
84	3	9
90	9	81
X̄ = 819, η = 10		
$\frac{810}{\eta}$ = 81		Total = 482

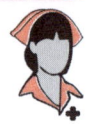

$$SD = \sqrt{\frac{\Sigma(X - \bar{X})^2}{\eta - 1}} = \sqrt{\frac{482}{10 - 1}}$$

$$= \sqrt{\frac{482}{9}} = \sqrt{53.55} = 7.31$$

So σ or SD = 7.31 for this data.

The meaning of standard can only be appreciated fully when we study it with reference to what is described as normal curve.

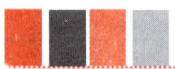
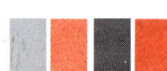

ASSESS YOURSELF

1. **What is the tabular presentation of data?**
2. **Write down the principles for designing a table from data.**
3. **What is graphic representation? Give rules for graphic representation.**
4. **Explain about the central tendency.**

Writing a Report

9

INTRODUCTION

Research report is the final and utmost outcome of the whole research process. Report writing is common to both academic and managerial situations.

In academics, reports are used for comprehensive and application oriented learning. It may be for the partial fulfillment of the degree courses. Student reports are called term papers, project reports, thesis or a dissertations. No research is complete unless the report is written and communicated. The researcher put out their initial finding in a research report, paper, monograph, which is later condensed into an article or expanded into a series of articles or a book. It is very necessary for the researcher to maintain the proper notes or the each step of the research progress so that these notes can be taken into consideration while preparing the research report.

CHARACTERISTICS OF A RESEARCH REPORT

A research report is the result of the researcher's hard work on the project. It should have the following characteristics:

❑   A research report must reflect its originality.

❑   A research report should be having the characteristic of conciseness to save the time and energy of the reader and force the writer to refine his ideas.

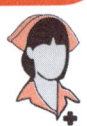

- It should have clarity to understand the points being made.
- Honesty is necessary to maintain the respect to the reader and the integrity of the author.
- The report should be full with the characteristics of completeness and accuracy so that the reader can take full use of it as desired.
- A research report must be long enough to cover the subject contents and short enough to maintain the interest among its users and consumers.
- The research report should solve the purpose for which the study is conducted.

CATEGORIES OF REPORT

Report mainly falls into three categories:

1. Information oriented reports.
2. Decision oriented reports.
3. Research oriented reports.

The substance and focus of the contents can determine the category however, a report may contain the characteristics of more than one category.

Information Oriented Reports

It describes any person, object, situation or concept. The following seven questions (6 Ws + 1 H) help to convey a comprehensive picture.

Subject	Action	Reason
Who	What	Why
Whom	When	
	Where	
	How	

Information reports are the first step to understand the existing situation for example epidemiology of disease, business, economics, technology. It helps to discuss and take decisions.

Decision Oriented Reports

These are the reports which adopt the problem solving approach steps:

- Identify the problem
- Constructing the criteria
- Generating and evaluating options
- Making a decision
- Drawing up action plan
- Working out to that plan

The decision reports are the difficult matters as they include a problem solving approach which helps only when one can question oneself again and again at every stage and bring to various thought processes to do a comprehensive analysis and synthesis.

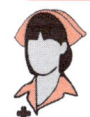

If the problem solving approach and steps are used merely as a form filling exercise, a superficial analysis and report will result.

A good decision report is structured sequentially but reflects comprehensively the iterative thinking process of decision makers.

Research Oriented Reports

Research reports contribute to the growth of subject literature. They pave the way for new information, significant hypothesis and innovative and rigorous methods of research and measurement. They broadly have the following organization:

- A problem
- Literature survey to find gaps in knowledge
- Nature and scope of study, hypothesis to be tested and significance and utility of study
- Methodology for collecting data, conducting the experiment, and analyzing the data
- Description and analysis of the experiment and data
- Findings, conclusions
- Recommendations and suggestions for further research
- Back up evidence and data

Most common type of the research reports are following:

- Thesis
- Research monograph
- Research article
- Newspaper magazine articles

FORMAT OF RESEARCH REPORT

The format of research report vary from institute to institute and university to university, however the basis contents of the report remains the same. Quantitative research reports typically follow a conventional formal referred as **IMRAD format.** It organizes the study material in four sections, i.e. Introduction, methods, results and discussion.

What so ever the format may be the researcher has to follow a proper sequence for their presentation and that study is divided into various sections.

- **Preliminary sections or front matter**
  - Title page
  - Approval sheet
  - Acknowledgement (If any)
  - Preface or foreword
  - Table of contents
  - List of tables and illustrations
- **Main body section**
  - Introduction
    - Statement of problem
    - Significance of problem
    - Purpose of study

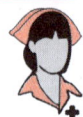

- o   Assumptions and delimitations
- o   Definitions of terms
- o   Hypothesis and assumptions underlying hypothesis
- Review of literature
- Study design/methodology
- Presentation and analysis of date
- Summary and conclusion
- Recommendations for further research
- **Reference section**
  - Bibliography
  - Appendix
  - Index

Preliminary Pages

Preliminary pages are the face pages of the thesis which give identification data of the researcher and the institute where research work has been done, completed and submitted.

Title page: It is the first page of the report. It should have all required information like identification data purpose and the problem of research. It should include the name of topic, full name of the researcher and his previous academic background, name of faculty/department where report submitted, etc.

An example of the title page is given below:

Title of the research study
Thesis submitted for the partial fulfillment of the degree in
Masters of Science in Nursing of BABA FARID UNIVERSITY, FARIDKOT IN
Year (20_____)
Name of the candidate
Name of the department and institute

- **Approval sheet:** It is the certification of the work from the guide/supervisor and the principal. This certifies that the candidate has conducted his study with full honesty and compassion. The signature of guide/supervision and principal are taken on this sheet.
- **Acknowledgement:** It is the gratitude and thanks of the people who have contributed their co-operation to complete the study. If the acknowledgement section is short it may be treated as the part of preface, if long then separate section may be made. At the end of the acknowledgement, only the author's name appears in italics in right hand corner.
- **Preface or foreword:** Preface or foreword is the pages in which the purpose of the study is mentioned and some part of acknowledgement. The preface is written by the author to indicate how the subject was chosen, its importance, need and focus. At the end of the preface, the authors name is given on the right side. On the left side address and place of writing the preface appear name, place, address and data are put in italics.
- **Table of contents:** In writing the table of contents, great care should be taken. The contents sheet is both summary and guide to the various segments of the book. The table of content should cover all essential parts of the book and yet be brief enough to be clear and attractive.

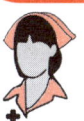

❑ **List of tables and illustrations:** List of tables and illustrations follow the table of contents. Each list starts on a separate page. If the items in each list are few, both the lists are put on same page but with different headings.

Only the first letter of the main words is capitalized in writing the titles of tables and illustrations.

The second and subsequent lines of an item are indented. The page number appears against first, second or third line where item description ends.

Tables and illustration are numbered continuously in serial order throughout the book in Arabic numbers (e.g. 1, 2, 3) or in decimal form (e.g. 1.1, 1.2, 1.3). In the latter classification, the first number refers to the chapter number and the second one to the serial of the table or illustration within the chapter.

Main Body Section

The main body of thesis or report is the very important part of the report writing. It starts from the statement of problem till the recommendations of the further studies.

Introduction

❑ It is the most important part of the research report from where one can make out the significance of the whole thing. The main purpose of the introduction is to discuss the background of the research project. In this section writer wants to presents his facts.

❑ **Statement of problem:** This section includes the statement of problem, its back ground, its significance and importance.

❑ **Purpose/significance and objectives of study:** This section lays the foundation on which the research study is based. It gives the basic answers for the questions like why this study is important? To whom is it important? And what is the benefit for it?

❑ **Hypothesis or assumptions:** Each research is based on a hypothesis or an assumption, which researchers have to test their research findings.

❑ **Scope and delimitation:** All studies have limitations and a finite scope. Limitations are often due to problems of time or money. The limitation section should deal with the question of bias and non-response precisely list of the limitations of the study. Describe the extent to which you believe the limitations degrade the quality of the research.

❑ **Operational definitions or definition of important terms:** These are the essential terms to the study or to use in a restricted or unusual manner, so that the reader may understand the concepts employed. This section involves the operationally defined terms used in the research study in the manner where researcher is going to study the variables.

Literature Review

As name indicates, it is related to the review of literature references to an extensive, exhaustive and systematic examination of publications relevant to research project. This chapter is important because it shows what previous researchers have explored and discovered about the phenomenon under study. If you are planning to explore a new area, the literature review should cite similar area of study or studies. The style for presenting the result of a literature review and analysis will vary according to the style requirement for courses, journals, thesis and dissertations, and grant proposals. However each of these style requires documentations of citations that support the statement that researcher make.

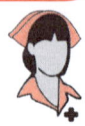

Study Design/Methodology

Methodology means to describe the method by which the study proceeds. It explains the design of study in detail. It includes:

- ❑ Design of research study
- ❑ Research setting
- ❑ Target population
- ❑ Sampling technique and sampling size
- ❑ Development and description of the research instrumentation
- ❑ Validity and reliability of research tools
- ❑ Procedure and time frame of data collection
- ❑ Pilot study
- ❑ Feasibility of study
- ❑ Ethical considerations
- ❑ Analysis plan

So from above we conclude that it gives an accurate detailed description about the work/study.

Presentation and Analysis of Data

This section can be presented in one or more chapters. All the data, which is collected, tabulated and statically analyzed should be given in this chapter. Description of study sample and analysis and interpretation of data through descriptive and inferential statistics and data usually presented through tables, graphs, pictures, etc.

Summary and Conclusion

This chapter includes the explanations of findings through critical analysis along with comparison with other similar research findings. This section also presents the verdict on whether these findings support the existing theories or not.

Conclusion includes the few paragraphs that summarize what you did and found. The present recommendations should be based on the findings.

The final limit of the report is written over in this chapter. The recommendations are also there.

Recommendations for the Further Research

Recommendations fall into two categories. The first is recommendations to the study sponsor. The second is recommendations for the other research. There is always a room for the improvement or refined the studies. What changes can be made if the same study is used again, etc.

Reference Section

This section follows the text section. First comes the bibliography then appendices and glossary and then index.

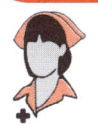

References/Bibliography

A bibliography contains the source of every reference cited in the any relevant work that the author has consulted. It gives the reader an idea of the literature available on the subject and that has influenced or aided the author.

The following information is given for each bibliography:

Books	Magazine/Newspaper
• Author/Authors	• Author/Authors

• Title
   ▪ Place of publication
   ▪ Publisher
   ▪ Date of publication
   ▪ Number of pages
	• Title of the article
	   ▪ Title of magazine
	   ▪ Volume number (Roman numerals)
	   ▪ Serial number (Arabic numerals)
	   ▪ Date of issue
	   ▪ Page number of the article

The bibliography should give a clear, complete description of the sources that were used while doing the research project and preparing the list.

Appendices

Supplementary and secondary references are put in the appendices section. This section help the author to authenticate the thesis and help the reader to check the data.

The materials usually put in the appendix are as below:

- Original data
- Long tables
- Long questions
- Supportive legal decisions, laws and documents
- Illustrative material
- Extensive computations
- Questionnaires and letters
- Schedules or forms used in collecting data
- Case studies histories
- Transcripts of interviews

Glossary

A glossary is the short dictionary giving definitions and examples of terms and phrases which are technical, used in special connotation by the author unfamiliar to reader or foreign to the language in which the book is written. It is listed as a major section in all capital letters in the table of contents.

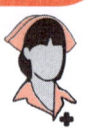

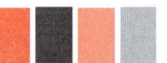 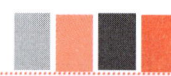

ASSESS YOURSELF

1. Explain characteristics of a research report.
2. What are the categories of report? Explain one in detail.
3. What is the importance of report writing in research? Give views.

Introduction to Statistics

10

Learning Objectives

- To know the uses and applications of statistics.
- To describe the classification of statistics.

Key Terms

- **Population:** Well-defined group of individuals being studied.
- **Unit:** Sampling unit as source of basic information.
- **Sample:** Representative of the entire population.
- **Variable:** Quality by which individuals differ among themselves.
- **Constant:** Quantity which does not vary.
- **Parameter:** Any numerical property.
- **Data:** Set of facts expressed in quantitative form.
- **Inference:** Conclusion about a population.
- **Accuracy:** Closeness of a computed value to its true value.
- **Precision:** Repeated measurements of the same quantity.

Statistic is a term used for how much or how many in a normal life. This means a measured or counted fact or piece of information stated as a figure such as height of one person, etc. "Statistics is the study of methods and procedures for collection, classification, analysis and interpretation of data to make scientific inferences from it".

The main characteristics of statistics are as follows:

- Statistic are aggregates of facts
- Statistics are always expressed numerically
- Statistics are influenced by multiplicity of causes
- Statistical data need to be collected in a systematic manner
- Statistical data is collected for a predetermined purpose
- Accuracy in collection of data is pre-empt.

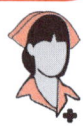

STATISTICAL TERMS

- **Population:** A group of study elements is called population or population refers to any well defined group of individuals who are being studied, or of observations of a particular type. For example, for the study of lung cancer the cigarette smokers may be the population.
- **Unit:** Smaller object or each individual of the population that can be investigated as the source of basic information. Units can be expressed as:
  - Sampling units during survey
  - Experimental units during experiments
- **Sample:** It is a group of sampling units, a portion of a population selected using a suitable method. It is regarded as the representative of the entire population.
- **Variables:** Variable is a quality which can vary from one individual to another. It is the characteristic by which individuals differ among themselves. The particular values of a variable are termed as variate. These variables are of mainly two types—quantitative and qualitative.
- **Constant:** Constant is a quantity which does not vary from one member of a group to another or within a particular set of defined conditions.
- **Parameter:** Parameter is any numerical property, characteristic that is descriptive of a population. Since parameters are descriptions of the population, a population can have many parameters.
- **Data:** Data is a set of facts expressed in quantitative form. It can be primary and secondary.
- **Inference:** It is simply a conclusion about a population. It can be of two types:
  1. Subject matter inference
  2. Statistical inference
- **Accuracy:** Accuracy is the closeness of a measured or computed value to its true value.
- **Precision:** Precision is the closeness of repeated measurements of the same quantity.

Statistics is a study that involves refining numerical and non-numerical information into the useful data. It is the game of numbers and the numbers are only which play essential role in statistics, as the numbers provide the raw material of statistics.

DEFINITIONS

We can define the statistics in many ways. According to Prof. Horace Secrist statistics means aggregate of facts affected to a marked extent by multiplicity of causes, numerically expressed, enumerated or estimated according to reasonable standards of accuracy, collected in a systematic manner for a predetermined purpose and placed in relation to each other.

According to Croxton and Cowden: Statistics is defined as collection, presentation, analysis and interpretation of numerical data.

USES AND APPLICATIONS

- It presents facts is definite form
- It facilitates comparisons
- It simplifies the masses of figures

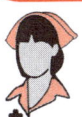

- ❑ It helps in formulating and testing hypothesis
- ❑ It helps in prediction
- ❑ Helps in collection, analysis and dissemination of various population health sciences
- ❑ Application of biostatistics in health sciences can be conceptualized properly.

CLASSIFICATION

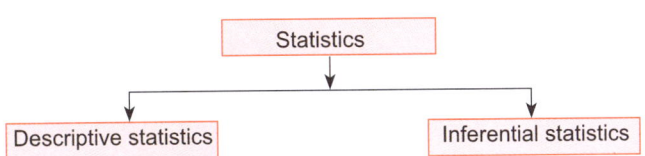

Statistics is broadly divided in two categories:

1. **Descriptive statistics:** It deals with enumeration, organization and graphical representation of data. For example, decennial census in India. This data is used to organize and summarize data to draw meaningful interpretations. Descriptive statistics also allow the researcher to interpret the data meaningfully, so that research questions can be answered completely and appropriately. Descriptive statistics may be categorized in several ways. Most simplified classification of the descriptive statistics include:
   - ■ Frequency distribution and graphical presentation
   - ■ Measurers of central tendency
   - ■ Measures of dispersion
   - ■ Measures of relationship

These all we had studied in detail in the chapter Analysis of Data.

2. **Inferential statistics** provides the procedure to draw an inference about the condition of that exist in a large set of observations. This branch of statistics is also known as sampling statistics. This is concerned with populations, and use sample data to make inference about the population or to test the hypothesis considered at the beginning of the research study. Inferential statistics help the researcher to determine if the difference found between two more groups, such as experimental and control group is a difference or only a chance difference that occurred because an unrepresentative sample was chosen from the population.

   Test of significance are the tests for the inferential statistics.

* These tests will be given in detail in chapter analysis of data unit.

STATISTICAL PACKAGES AND APPLICATIONS

Traditionally, in the field of health care biostatistics, data has been handled manually. It involves more money, material and man power. It needs much time and as it is done manually, results take more time and will have different types of errors. The advent of computers and their popularity changed the way. Biostatistics is now applied to health sciences. Computer hardware and appropriate software have optimized the various processes involved in the application of biostatistics by making the data analysis and storage easier, faster and errorless. On the other

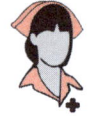

hand it has also improved the comprehension of data through the use of sophisticated graphic presentation techniques.

As all the coins have two sides, the same way with the number of advantages of using the computer in statistics there are few disadvantages also. The usefulness of results only depends upon the statistical competence of the user.

There are a number of computer packages available to be used for the statistical analysis. Commonly packages used in statistical analysis are as follows:

- ❑ Microsoft Excel
- ❑ Statistical package for social sciences (SPSS)
- ❑ Statistical analysis system (SAS)
- ❑ Minitab
- ❑ Sites for Minitab are *www.mintab.com.*

ASSESS YOURSELF

1. What are the uses and applications of statistics?
2. Explain the role of computer in statistics.

Utilization of Research Findings

11

Learning Objectives

- To communicate the research findings.
- To utilize the research findings.

Key Terms

- **Utilization:** Used knowledge generated through research to guide.
- **Communication of research findings:** Developing a research report and disseminating to a variety of audiences with presentations and publications.
- **Research findings:** Final findings of research.

Nursing is considered as both art and science, so research is a necessary part of nursing. Florence Nightingale was the first nurse who not only conducted the research, but also the first to disseminate research findings and implement research based practice.

Today after almost more than 100 years, the need of research based on traditional rather than science. In today's cost and time conscious health care environment, nurses cannot afford to spend time on unnecessary or ineffective procedures. At times when nurses are now asked to take care of most complicated illness and demanding patients, striving for decreased length of stay, the nurse must work smarter, not only harder. Although many different reasons are put forward for the research-practice gap, there is agreement that way should be found to strengthen the role of research in nursing and to overcome the factors inhabiting role.

There are certain barriers in utilizing the nursing research which are to be seen and solved.

BARRIERS IN UTILIZATION OF NURSING RESEARCH

Funk, Champagne, Wiese and Tornquist (1991) identified the barriers to research utilization under four categories. They are:

1. Factors related to nurses.
2. Nursing research factors.
3. Organizational factors.
4. Communication factors.

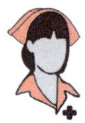

Factors Related to Nurses

❑ Nurses have lack of time, motivation, confidence, research knowledge and resources
❑ Nurses do not see the value of research for practice
❑ They see little benefit for self from research
❑ They are inflexible and unwilling to change/try new ideas
❑ They are not documented need to change practice
❑ Nurses lack confidence in new research findings
❑ Nurses do not feel capable of evaluating the quality of the research
❑ Nurses lack time and resources to stay in touch with knowledgeable colleagues with whom to discuss the research
❑ Nurses are unaware about the importance of the research.

Factors Related to Nursing Research

❑ The research has methodological inadequacies
❑ The conclusions drawn from the research are not justified
❑ The research has not been replicated
❑ The literature reports conflicting results
❑ The nurses are uncertain whether to believe the results of the research
❑ Research reports/articles are not published fast enough
❑ Nursing research generally lack the appropriate clinical applicable recommendations

Organizational Factors

❑ Organizations failed to provide access to journals and research resources
❑ Organizations lack the funding to support new research findings
❑ Administration does not allow implementation of new research findings
❑ Physicians will not cooperate with implementation of new research findings
❑ There is insufficient time on the job to implement new ideas
❑ Other staff is not supportive of implementation
❑ The facilities are inadequate for implementation
❑ Nurses do not feel that they have enough authority to change patient care procedures
❑ Nurses do not have time to read research literature and participate in research activities
❑ The nurses feel results are not generalized to their settings.

Communication Factors

❑ Lack of collaboration between researcher and clinicians
❑ Lack of presentation of research findings to nurses in clinical setting
❑ Lack of publication in clinical nursing journals
❑ Lack of understandable research publications
❑ Overwhelming amount of contradicting information in medical and nursing journals as well as in textbooks

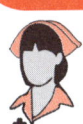

- Implication for practice are not made clear
- Research reports/articles are not readily available
- The research is not reported clearly and readably
- Statistical analyses are not understandable
- The relevant literature is not compiled in one place
- The research is not relevant to the nurses practice.

APPLICATION OF NURSING RESEARCH

- Promote basic knowledge for infrastructure management which includes drug treatment, nursing or medical management of disease or health care or nursing care referred.
- Developments of new tools, which may be drugs, vaccines. Diagnostic tools are operative technique.
- Research provides the data for better management of scarce resources and can guide health policies and actions.
- The unique function of the nurse is to assist the individual sick or well in the performance of those activities contributing to health, its recovery that the client would perform unaided if he had the necessary strength, will or knowledge, and to do this in such a way as to help the client gain independence as rapidly as possible.

    Three essential components of professional nursing are care, cure and coordination. The care aspect is more than to take 'care of', it is also 'caring for' and 'caring about'. It is dealing with human being under stress, frequently over long periods of time. It is providing comfort and support in time of anxiety, loneliness and helplessness. It is listening, evaluating and intervening appropriately.

    The expending role of the nurse demands research to provide a wide philosophical base for health care to stimulate interest in research and to increase the pool of potential researchers.

- Provision of a caring relationship that facilitates health and healing
- Integration of objective data with knowledge gained from an appreciation of the patient or group subjective experience
- Attention to the range of human experiences and responses to health and illness within the physical and social environment
- Application of scientific knowledge to this process of diagnosis or treatment through the use of judgment and critical thinking
- Advancement of professional nursing knowledge through scholarly research
- Influence of social and public policy to promote social justice.

    So concluding with certain changes in profession, the utilization of the research can be done.

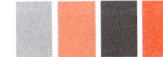

ASSESS YOURSELF

1. What is the importance of utilization of research findings?
2. What are the barriers in utilization of nursing research?
3. What are the applications of nursing research?

Notes

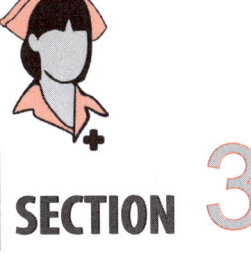

SECTION 3

PROFESSIONAL TRENDS AND ADJUSTMENT

- ➲ Nursing: A Profession

- ➲ Professional Ethics

- ➲ Personal and Professional Development

- ➲ Legislation in Nursing

- ➲ Professional and Related Organizations

Nursing: A Profession

12

- To describe a profession.
- To discuss about nursing, nurse and nursing profession.

Key Terms

- **Profession:** An occupation with ethical components that is devoted to human and social welfare.
- **Monasteries:** Where monks and nuns, worked as nurses to protect the needy people.
- **Deaconesses:** Those who are doing religious teachings.

Nursing in India has strived hard in the past to meet the criteria and now has become a recognized profession. This is evident by higher qualifications required for admission in nursing education, better and reasonably adequate salaries and fringe benefits offered. Nursing in India has certainly become essential profession and very important and vital to society. Nursing profession is meeting all other criteria except the autonomy in true sense. However, professional nursing organizations and nursing leaders are trying to become more and more autonomous in formulating policies and control on their professionals.

DEFINITION

The dictionary meaning of profession is vocation, calling, especially one which involves some branch of learning or service as a learned profession of divinity law, medicine, etc.

Profession is defined as an occupation with ethical components, that is devoted to the promotion of human and social welfare.

The services offered by a profession are based on specialized knowledge and skills that have been developed in a scientific and learned manner.

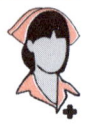

CHARACTERISTICS/CRITERIA

A criteria is the scale on which we can measure the characteristics of a thing that gives us a clear picture. The criteria for a profession can be discussed as follows:

- Profession is a form of employment especially one that is respected in society as honorable and is possible only for an educated person and after training in some special branch of knowledge.
- A profession has its own body of knowledge based on social and scientific principles.
- The members of a profession utilize this knowledge to identify and solve problems.
- A profession has service aim as well as academic and theoretical aim. The services offered by a profession are in response to the needs of the society and are fundamental to the promotion of human and social welfare.
- A profession constantly enlarges its body of knowledge through research in order to improve its services to the society.
- A profession determines the qualifications necessary for those who enter into practice.
- A profession has a code of ethics.
- A profession recognizes its responsibilities to develop institutions in order to offer specialized study and practice required to learn methods of service and develop skills for the better service of the society.

It is important to remember that above criteria enables to judge and evaluate the profession and helps to improve it. The above criteria could be summarized in a few words. A profession should be:

- Intellectual
- Scientific
- Requires higher education
- Essential
- Self-governing
- Service oriented
- Provides personal development and economic security for members.

NURSING AS PROFESSION

Historically, only medicine, law and engineering were accepted as professions. Today 'professional' is a term commonly used to identify many types of people ranging from wrestlers and rock stars, to call professionals. Nursing in India has strived hard in the past to meet the criteria and now comes to be recognized as a profession. This is evident by higher qualifications required for admission in nursing education better and reasonably adequate salaries and fringe benefits offered. More means of economic security are available. Members are taking up research. The increasing numbers of nursing educational programs have been added, institutions of higher learning in nursing and introduction of university and post basic courses in nursing etc. are witness.

Nursing in India has certainly become essential profession and very important and vital to society. Nursing profession is meeting all other criteria except the autonomy in true sense. The criteria of autonomy to the profession on self-governing has not yet attained that status. It is still considered as allied to medicine.

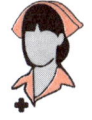

However, professional nursing organizations and nursing leaders are trying to become more and more autonomous in formulating policies and control on their professional activities.

We certainly have a well-organized and well defined body of knowledge based upon scientific principles looked at the intellectual level of higher learning.

Research and scientific approach have to be implemented in nursing practice and nursing education.

PROFESSIONAL NURSE AND EDUCATIONAL PREPARATION

Professional nurse is a graduate of a recognized nursing school who has fulfilled the requirements for a registered nurse in a state in which she is licensed to practice.

Candidates who satisfy the basic requirements are selected by the authority to undergo the training in a recognized school or college of nursing. They complete the basic course of study according to the prescribed syllabus approved by the Indian Nursing Council and by the State Council. The length of the period of training version with the type of program. After the successful completion of the course, the candidate receives a diploma or a bachelor's degree in nursing.

The subjects in the nursing curriculum are grouped as follows:

- **Physical and biological sciences**
  - Anatomy and physiology
  - Microbiology and pathology
  - Physics and chemistry
  - Nutrition
  - Computer application
- **Social sciences**
  - Psychology and sociology
  - History of nursing, professional adjustment and management
- **Medical sciences**
  - Medicine and surgery
  - Pediatrics and obstetrics
  - Materia medica
  - Psychiatry
- **Nursing sciences**
  - Medical and surgical nursing
  - Obstetrics and gynecological nursing
  - Pediatric nursing
  - Psychiatric nursing
  - Community health nursing
  - Fundamentals of nursing
  - Advance nursing
  - Research in nursing

EVOLUTION OF NURSING

Nursing has been called the oldest of arts and the youngest of the professions. Nursing has been involved in the existing culture, shaped by it and yet helping to develop it. The history of nursing

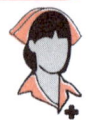

has been that of frustration, ignorance and misunderstanding. It is a great turning point in the world progress has also been the important turning points in the history of nursing.

Contemporary nursing practice requires a combination of intellectual achievement, ethical standards, scientific knowledge, technical skills and personal compassion. Gradually, over the centuries, these elements have evolved and blended together. During this evolutionary process nursing practice has been influenced by external factors such as economics, religion, politics, scientific advances, wars and changing life style.

To see the evolution of nursing we can have the historic view of nursing to the modern nursing. We can divide it in the following cases:

❑ Early Christian Ear (1–500 AD)
❑ Early Middle Ages (500–1000 AD)
❑ Late Middle Ages (1000–1500 AD)
❑ Modern Nursing

Early Christian Era (1 AD to 500 AD)

This era is known as the pre Christian times and was influenced by most religious beliefs. According to that era disease was accepted as punishment by the God. Then Jesus Christ brought a new aspect that of thoughtful interest in others and to develop the helping attitude. We has a good record of nursing of this era. Apostolic orders of women were taken. The three type of men or women assisted in the work of Church. They were:

1. Deaconesses (those who are doing religious teachings).
2. A second order of widows.
3. The virgin.

The first type *deaconesses* did teachings and preachings and care for their sicks in their homes.

Widows also assisted deaconesses with their work in home visiting and caring the sick people.

The third type virgin are the younger women assisted in caring for the Church vestments and giving out alms to poor.

Then almost in 4th century deaconesses order disappear and widows and virgins interested in religious works went to monasteries as nuns and continue the nursing services.

In Rome women of high rank, had much freedom. As Christian they become interested in works of charity and nursing. Some wealthy women formed organized groups. They establish monasteries, hospitals and other facilities for sick people. These places became heaven for many homeless sick or orphan people when the empire of Rome destroyed.

Early Middle Ages (500 AD to 1000 AD)

Early middle age is considered as the dark age in the history of medicine and nursing. The beginning of this era was with the fall of Roman Empire and the Roman was destroyed. People become homeless, sick and helpless. There was hue and cry all over. Roman authorities shifted their capital.

At that crucial time these protective units were developed. They were:

❑ The monasticism
❑ The feudalism
❑ The guilds

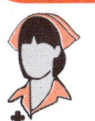

Monasticism

Monasticism means life, rules, condition of monasteries where monks and nuns lived so they protect and help the needy people of society. Nuns and monks worked as nurses.

Feudalism and guilds were the agricultural and treaders people, they help to run monasteries and help in nursing areas through economy.

Late Middle Ages (1000 AD to 1500 AD)

This was the period of military orders. Religious was between Muslims and Christians lasted nearly 200 years.

In this era industrial and political revolutions take place. Medical, nursing, etc. books were published. The interest and belief of the people to the medical and nursing sciences changes. New hospitals were built in 17th to middle of 19th century.

Although new hospitals were built but it was a dark period for nursing, as during this period the nurses were poorly fed, over worked, lacking in skills and morals, doing only cleaning, laundry and scrubbing. Then the modern nursing emerges.

Modern Nursing

Progress in science and medicine during past three centuries increased interest for better nursing services and nursing training. As days advanced, it became evident that love and care alone were not sufficient to promote health and overcome disease. Skill, expertise and knowledge become essential for nursing. As science advanced the emphasis on knowledge emerged, knowledge of facts and scientific principles provide initiating force for nursing to become profession.

Then the era of modern nursing commences with the work of Florence Nightingale the founder of modern nursing.

She was born on May 12, 1820. She succeeded to a great extent to improve health laws to reform hospitals to recognize military medical services and establish nursing as a profession with two missions.

Nursing in Sickness and Health

After Crimean War, she served on several commissions and wrote about health sanitation, hospitals and nursing education. In 1860 she established a school at St. Thomas Hospital and gives the principles, which are as follows:

- ❑ Nurses should have practice training in hospital setup
- ❑ Nurses should live in a home to form their moral character and discipline
- ❑ Nursing education must be directed by a nurse
- ❑ Nursing education is necessary for a nurse because she must know the reason why she is to teach others
- ❑ Theory and practice must be correlated
- ❑ The school should be economically independent.

Towards the end of 19th century, "Nightingale nurses" provided leadership and set a pattern which is the basis of nursing education today.

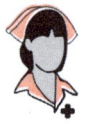

NURSING PROFESSION IN INDIA

Nurses were recruited in India for the first time in 1914, being attached to the queen Alexandra's military nursing service. East India Company started their hospitals in Madras.

Nurses were brought from England to be incharge and first six students were those who had previously received their diplomas in midwifery.

Later this plan was reversed. General training was taken first followed by the course of midwifery.

❑ **In 1891:** Bai Kashibai Ganpat was the first Indian nurse to come for training. Miss TK Andra Nirala was an outstanding graduate of the JJ group of hospitals. She worked hard to raise the status of nursing profession in India and has given much of her time to the interest of Indian Nurses Association of Illinois (INAI).

❑ **1907–1910:** The North India united board of examiners for mission hospitals was organized and set up rules for admissions and standards of training and conducted a public examination.

❑ **In 1913:** The first nursing examination was held by source India Board.

❑ **In 1926:** A mid India Board formed. A nursing council constituted in Chennai.

❑ **By 1939:** All states except Assam had a nursing council board for the purpose of carrying out similar functions.

❑ **1949:** The Indian nursing council was constituted with the object of establishing a uniform standard of nursing in the country.

❑ **1952:** First 10 months course in a public health nursing.

❑ **1946:** University education for nurses at the college of nursing Vellore and New Delhi.

❑ **1973:** Punjab university two colleges of nursing at Chandigarh and Ludhiana to introduce BSc Nursing Program.

❑ **1960:** University of Delhi introduces a course for MSc Nursing. Then the PhD in nursing is started. The Raj Kumari Amrit Kaur College of Nursing, New Delhi has established a department of nursing research in co-operation with WHO. As the days passes the professionalism of nursing shinning day-by-day.

QUALITIES/CHARACTERISTICS OF PROFESSIONAL NURSE

A professional nurse is a graduate of a recognized nursing school who has met the requirements for a registered nurse in a state in which she is licensed to practice. Nursing as a career which calls for certain special qualities. According to Miss Florence Nightingale characteristics of a nurse should be: "Nurse should be no gossip, no vain talker—be strictly sober and honest; but more than this she must be a devoted women, she must have a respect for calling—she must be a sound, a close and a quick observer and she must be a woman of delicate and decent feeling".

Some essential qualities of a nurse are as follows:

❑   Love for the fellow human beings

❑   Honesty and loyalty

❑   Discipline and obedience

❑   Alertness and intelligent observation

❑   Technical competence

- ☐ Dependability and adjustability
- ☐ Ability to inspire confidence
- ☐ Resourcefulness
- ☐ Economy of time, material and energy
- ☐ Courtesy and dignity
- ☐ Sympathy
- ☐ Empathy
- ☐ Fact and poise
- ☐ Intelligence and common sense
- ☐ Patience
- ☐ Sense of humor
- ☐ Good physical health
- ☐ Sound mental health
- ☐ Generosity
- ☐ Gentleness and quietness

She should have the qualities of the literal meaning of a NURSE. These are:

- ☐ **N**–Nobility, knowledge
- ☐ **U**–Usefulness, understanding
- ☐ **R**–Righteousness, responsibility
- ☐ **S**–Simplicity, sympathy
- ☐ **E**–Efficiency, equanimity

ROLES OF A PROFESSIONAL NURSE

In the past the principle role of nurses was to provide care and comfort as they come out specific nursing function. The contemporary nurses function in the interrelated roles of the following:

- ☐ **Care giver:** A nurse meets the client's holistic health care needs to promote health and the healing process. The nurse provides treatment for specific disease and applies measures to restore the emotional and social well-being of the client. She preserves the dignity of the client.
- ☐ **Advocate:** A nurse protects the client from kind of injuries. The nurse assists the clients in expressing their rights whenever necessary. The nurse also works to preserve the client's legal and human rights in time of health illness and during the process of dying. The nurse advocates the clients right in general way by keeping in mind the clients religion and culture.
- ☐ **Critical thinker:** Nurse uses decision making and critical thinking skills in conjunction with the nursing process.
- ☐ **Teacher:** The nurse provides her clients, their family members and other members of the society with information about health treatment or therapy and life style changes. She determines that the client fully understood. She gives health education on diet, about preventive measures of disease.
- ☐ **Communicator:** Effective communication is an essential element of all professions including nursing. For effective nursing practice, open and consistent communication is vital.

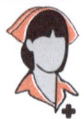

As a communicator, nurse provide information to other health team members about planned and unplanned nursing care through documentation, reports and verbally.

❑ **Manager:** Nurse manages and coordinates client care, supervises and guides the client in rehabilitative activities related to daily living. She can also be an effective manager at various level of administration. She manages nursing care of not only of one patient in hospital but also families and in communities. She delegates the nursing activities to auxiliary workers and other nurses.

❑ **Researcher:** Nurse participates in research works related to health care. A nurse researcher usually conducts studies and investigates problems to improve client's health and nursing care. She does many quantitative and qualitative researches.

❑ **Rehabilitation:** Nurse ensures that the client returns to a maximal state of functioning. Rehabilitation is a process by which individual's returns to maximal levels of functioning after illness, accident or other events.

Rehabilitative and restorative care activities ranges from teaching clients to walk with crutches, to help the client to cope with life style changes often associated with chronic illness.

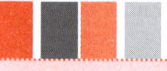 **ASSESS YOURSELF**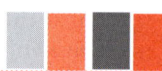

1. Define profession, write down the criteria for nursing profession.

2. Discuss nursing as profession.

3. Write down the qualities of a professional nurse.

4. What are the roles of a professional nurse?

Professional Ethics

Learning Objectives

- To discuss about the profession ethics and etiquettes.
- To describe about the role of nurse.
- To describe about the evolution of nursing.

Key Terms

- Ethics
- Etiquettes
- Resigning: Quitting the job by own wish.

MEANING AND RELATIONSHIP OF PROFESSIONAL ETHICS AND ETIQUETTES

Professional Ethics

Ethics word comes from the Greek word 'ethos' means customs and guiding belief. It means a code of moral behavior. These are the rules or principles that govern right conduct. They deal with what is good and bad, with moral duty and obligation. Hence, we can say that code of ethics will state what kind of behavior is expected from the members of a profession. In nursing profession code of ethics provide professional standards for nursing activities which protect nurse and client.

Professional Etiquettes

Etiquettes are the code of good manners that a nurse should follow. As a nurse one should follow some essential good manners/etiquettes as follows:

- Nurse should be courteous, gentle and polite in talks to all
- Greet your seniors, co-workers, patients, clients with appropriate words according to time of the day, e.g. Good morning, good evening, etc.
- Address the seniors with respect and proper title like madam, sister, etc.
- Stand up when people with higher rank enter your room, offer them a decent sitting place
- Stand up when answering questions in classroom

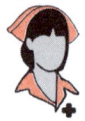

- Open the door for the seniors and stand aside for them to pass
- Excuse yourself when overtaking a senior person
- Stand aside and give way to seniors, when you cross them on the way, e.g. in the corridors, on stair cases etc.
- Maintain silence wherever and whenever necessary, e.g. classroom, library, studyroom and dormitories
- Keep the dress neat and tidy
- While on duty never use any form of jewellery, that may interfere with work
- Obey seniors without arguing
- Help the seniors to carry a heavy load if you find them on the way
- Say 'thank you' when someone is doing a favor for you and also when someone corrects you
- Be punctual always
- Get prior permission from the sister in charge before you take any article from any department
- Avoid thumb sucking and nail biting
- Do not delay the answers to the questions. Give the answer immediately and appropriately
- In the assembly let the seniors take the first seat
- Keep eye contact and sit face to face when listening to some one
- Say 'excuse me' even if you hurt others accidentally
- Never let others secret go out of you
- Knock at door and wait for the answer before you enter into other room
- Cover your mouth when you cough or sneeze
- Excuse yourself before you interfere with others engaged in talking or doing some work
- One should not give or receive any gift or present especially from the clients and their relatives.

Relationship of Professional Ethics and Etiquettes

Nurses should have the ethics and professional etiquettes both as these are two sides of one job. It eliminates professional ethical dilemmas and help in ethical, decision making. It helps in caring commands fidelity oneself and guards the right and privilege of the nurse to act in keeping with an informed moral conscience. It is not possible in real life to separate ethical behavior from all other behaviors and actions. Every action of ours can be judged as a moral action or otherwise. The nursing profession uses code for nurses, "Ethical concepts applied to nursing" as its guides for professional conduct. Hence professional ethics and etiquettes go side by side and complete each other.

Code of Ethics for Nurses

Ethics are the rules or principles that govern right conduct. They deal with what is good and bad, and with moral duty and obligations. Ethics are designed to protect the rights of human beings. Ethics are characteristics of a profession and are called a code. In nursing, code of ethics provides professional standards for nursing activities which protect the nurse and the client.

Some of the standards given in the code of ethics for nurse are also stated in the Nightingale pledge given earlier.

In 1973 the International Council of Nursing (ICN) adopted the code of ethics as follows:

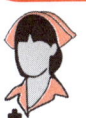

ICN Code of Ethics for Nurses (1973)

The fundamental responsibility of the nurse is four fold:

1. To promote health.
2. To prevent illness.
3. To restore health.
4. Alleviate suffering

- The need for nursing is universal; inherent in nursing is respect for life, dignity and rights of man. It is unrestricted by consideration of nationality, race, creed, color, age, sex, politics or social status.
- Nurses render health services to the individual, the family, and the community and coordinate their services with those related groups.

Nurses and People

- The nurses primary responsibility is to those people who require nursing care
- The nurse in providing care, promotes an environment in which the values, customs and spiritual beliefs of the individual are respected
- The nurse holds confidence personal information and uses judgment in sharing their information.

Nurses and Practices

- The nurse carries personal responsibility for nursing practice and for maintaining competence by continual learning
- The nurse uses judgment in relation to individual competence when accepting and delegating responsibility
- The nurse when acting in a professional capacity should at all times maintain standards of personal conduct which reflects credit upon the profession.

Nurses and Society

The nurses shares with other citizens the responsibility for initiating and supporting action to meet health and social needs of the public.

Nurses and Co-workers

- The nurses sustains a cooperative relationship with co-workers in nursing and other fields
- The nurse takes appropriate action to safeguard the individual when it care endangered by a co-worker or any other person.

Nurses and Profession

- The nurse plays a major role in determining and implementing desirable standards of nursing practice and nursing education
- The nurse is active in developing a care of professional knowledge
- The nurse acting through the professional organization participates in establishing and maintaining equitable social and economic working conditions in nursing.

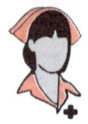

Ethical Principles

Ethical principles actually control professionalism, nursing practice much more than to ethical theories. Principles encompass basic promises from which rules are developed. Ethical principles that nurse should consider when making decisions are as follows:

- Respect for persons
- Respect for autonomy
- Respect for freedom
- Respect for beneficence (Doing good)
- Respect for nonmaleficence (Avoiding harm to others)
- Respect for veracity
- Respect for justice (Fair and equal treatment)
- Respect for rights
- Respect for fidelity
- Confidentiality

Nightingale Pledge

I solemnly pledge myself before God
And in the presence of this assembly
To pass my life in purity
And to practice my profession faithfully
I will abstain from whatever is deleterious and mischievous
And will not take or knowingly administer any harmful drug
I will do all in my power to maintain
And elevate the standard of my profession
And will hold in confidence
All personal matters committed to my keeping
And all family affairs coming to my knowledge
In the picture of my calling
With loyalty I will endeavor to aid the physician in his work
And devote myself to the welfare of those committed to my care.

Etiquettes for Employment

Employment is the first step to enter in profession, for serving the profession while entering into any profession, we should have a knowledge what to do, how to do, where to do and from where we get the information.

Locating a Position

For the employment one should know how to see a position which I wish to join when a person has chosen nursing as a field of career we should try to get information about particular kinds of positions we can love.

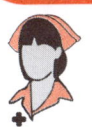

We can get information through:

❑ **Nursing journals:** The advertisements are given in the nursing journals by the institutions or employing authorities. There are a number of national and international journals available. So the position can be taken within the country or over. These advertisements include the desired qualifications and the salary benefits, address and their contact numbers.

❑ **Newspapers:** Other source of information is newspaper where the advertisements are given and considered. It is the biggest source and easily and cheaply available.

❑ **Direct contact with institution:** This is the way when the institutional personal are known to you or the employees are known to the person and this helps in position. One can decide to choose one that suits the qualification, personality and experience.

❑ **Pamphlets, radio, television, internet, etc.:** All other medias may help in choosing a position to which you can apply easily and can have the position.

When you have become interested in a particular position and wish to apply, you should try to secure further information regarding, working hours, quantity and quality of work, prospectus of position and promotion allowances, size of institution, management and other benefits by writing or interview before you make a final decision.

Applying and Accepting a Position

To apply for a job: There are there methods for this:

1. If you are already holding position somewhere it is always necessary to inform your employer that you are applying for the other position. It may be through the letter or application.

2. Writing a letter or application to the institute is a way to apply for the position. Check the last date. It may be an online application or a simple hard copy application.

3. To apply a job, the institute may have organized a prescribed application form which should be filled online or on papers.

One should be very particular about the application form. The letter of application can be a picture to project your image to institute. The application letter should be seen for the paper you use, the form of the letter, the standard of English or the other language used, neatness and legibility of your writing. All represent your standards as a person and as a member of a profession.

If the names and references of some persons are necessary first take the permission of the person whose name and address is given to the institution. It is also courteous to inform those who give references about the result of your application.

A personal interview may be required by employer for the selection for a position can be finalized.

Personal Interviews

A personal interview is valuable for both aspirant employ and employer. The personal meeting leads to evaluate the person directly as person as natural appearance, abilities and personality. It gives many questions which are difficult to ask by writing.

It helps the person to evaluate the place and the people with whom you are going to work.

One should prepare oneself carefully for the interview as already explained it gives the impression of yourself. And sometimes first impression is the last impression. Some suggestions are given as follows as to prepare yourself for an interview:

❑ Confirm the date, time and place

❑ Reach the place of interview well before time or spot the place one day prior to the interview. It will relieve last minute anxiety.

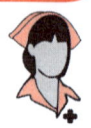

- ❑ Carry with your necessary documents. Make them ready with xerox copies
- ❑ Be ready with complete personal information and with your own questions
- ❑ Put on attractive, sensible and descent dress according to the position applied for
- ❑ Try to feel relax and behave naturally
- ❑ Try to practice an interview with friend or in front of mirror, if possible
- ❑ Be honest and straight forward in your conversation and look directly at the interviewer when you speak
- ❑ Do not criticize present job or employer or co-workers
- ❑ Do not express your feeling for example desire for position or disappointment if rejected.

Accepting the Job

When all the procedure for information of job, applying for job, and interviewing for job, all the conditions and positions are favorable, the person can accept the job. An appointment letter will be sent to the candidate by the employing authority, giving you date of appointment, designation, salary, allowances and the time and date of reporting for duty, on the given data. If due to any reason you are unable to accept the job or join the job on the given date, then the authority should be intimate immediately.

Appointment Letter

Address   Date _____

....

....

Dear ....

Further to our offer letter dated... .we are pleased to appoint you as in our hospital on the following terms and conditions.

a) You will be on probation upto.....................months. Thereafter if services are found satisfactory, your services will be confirmed.

b) Your pay scale is RS .... and you will get Rs ....PM. as basic pay

c) You will be entitled to get leaves and medical benefits according to institution rules.

d) You will be expected to abide by the hospital rules and regulations in force from time to time

e) You will be a full time employee of the hospital and are not allowed to work anywhere else.

Yours sincerely

Administrator

I have gone through my job description and accept it fully.

_____
Signature of employee

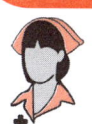

Success in a Position

After accepting a position in job the success is the aim of the personal and professional. It is important for the own satisfaction and the standard of work. If the position is of the choice and interest, it is likely you will be highly motivated to do the best and can carry professional responsibilities.

Interest in work, attitude towards work has an influential impact on the success. The necessity to change the position will come at some point in the career when it became necessary to change the position one should know how it is to be done.

Resigning a Position

Sometime due to many reasons one cannot continue the job like personal and family circumstances, promotion, going on for higher education, or just a desire for change.

The letter of resignation should be written in a professional manner, on a white sheet, expressing in a polite, honest and objective manner your reason for leaving.

Proper notification is professional and important. A notice of one month or three month according to norms of institute should be considered sufficient and reasonable unless it is not an emergency.

Although it is assured that all professional nursing persons should learn the approved methods of applying, accepting and resigning from a position. It is seen they have not frequently observed rules. It is however, necessary to know and practice the necessary etiquettes.

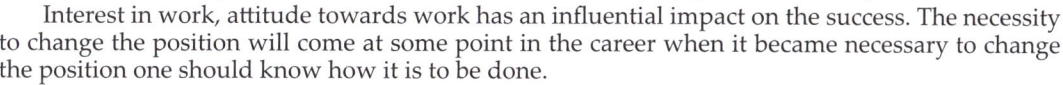

Joining Letter

Date..................................

The Personal Manager,

....

....

Subject: Joining letter

Sir,

I thank you very much for your letter dated .... offering me appointment for the post of.................................

I am joining my duty today dated...(Fornoon/afternoon)

My present Address and telephone no.

....

....

_____

Signature of employee

Designation ....

Department ....

_____

Signature of employee

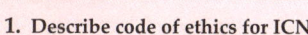

ASSESS YOURSELF

1. Describe code of ethics for ICN.
2. What are the ethical principles?
3. Learn and recite Nightingale pledge, discuss the meaning of it.

14 Personal and Professional Development

Learning Objectives

- To define and discuss about continuing education in nursing.
- To know about futuristic nursing.
- To describe the career in nursing.

Key Terms

- **Continue education:** Education after the completion of basic education.
- **Orientation:** Act required to let the others know about the area or things.
- **Development:** The process of changing in a positive way to advance form.

CONTINUING EDUCATION

Introduction

Continuing nursing education is a modern implicative, it must be future oriented geared to facing new situations and to the making of new responses appropriate for these situations. Continuing education programs should be developed by nurses and conducted within nursing or in general education system in cooperation with nurses. This program helps to keep nurses alert and interested in her profession.

Definitions

Continuing education is all the learning activities that occur after an individual has completed his basic education.

—**Cooper**

That education which builds on previous education.

—**Shannon**

Meaning and Importance

Continuing education in nursing consists of systematic learning experiences designed to enlarge the knowledge and skills of nurses as distinct from education towards an academic degree or preparing as a beginning professional practitioner, continuing professional education activities have more specific content applicable to the individual. Immediate goals are generally of shorter

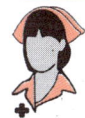

duration, sponsored by college, universities, health agencies and professional organizations and may be conducted in variety of settings.

Some of the important features and importance of continuing education are as following:

- Unified approach
- Relationships with other systems
- Comprehensiveness
- Accessibility for women health workers
- Integration with management process
- Analysis of needs as a basis for learning continuity
- Internally coordinated
- Relevance in planning
- Credibility and economic
- Appropriateness in implementations

Scope, Need and Opportunities

- For career advancement
- To ensure the safe and effective nursing care with new technology
- To meet the needs of population and we should cater the need of services
- To meet the changing in roles, concept and society, as new knowledge and technologies emerge
- To acquire specialized skills of personnel and meet technological adjuncts
- Nurses with research aptitude and preparation are needed
- To meet the demand for specialized nursing services
- To meet the health needs of public expectations
- Recruitment functions
- Recognize gaps in their knowledge
- Eagerness to fill the gap in knowledge and skill
- To improve communication between participants, faculty, community and health sector
- Shape or support the university educational policies and practices
- To ensure quality of education
- To maintain, educational, academic and clinical standards, continuing education program contributes to the development of 3 domains and leadership, management for the nurses. These skills are very helpful as the nurse is expected to function with the help of auxiliary personnel in her working condition. Her competence is very much needed. Continued education program should be conducted at a time of the day when the ward work is lightest and large number of staff can attend. This continuing education program helps to keep nurses alert and interested in her profession.

CAREER IN NURSING

Nursing in India has strived hard in past to meet the criteria and comes to be recognized as profession. Earlier the nurse means only a person giving care to the sick in the hospital. Now with the changes, vast opportunities are available for a nurse to develop her career in nursing. Wider

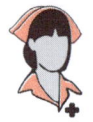

range of opportunities for a nurse for service are available according to the education, i.e. whether the nurse in ANM, GNM, Basic graduate, post basic graduate, having specialization certificates or having super specialization in various fields. The nurse may choose the field of her practice within the country or in abroad. Due to some following seasons the nursing services have been influenced and resulted in increasing the need for nurses and varieties of services.

- ❑ International trends in nursing profession and nursing education
- ❑ Awareness of the health needs by the society has developed
- ❑ Economic conditions for nursing services has been improving
- ❑ Population trends of the country is changing
- ❑ Need for specialization because of forgoing points
- ❑ Fast growing new developments in medicine and medical practice
- ❑ New knowledge and procedures developed through research in science in general. Nowadays scientific progress is so rapid that it is difficult to keep pace with it
- ❑ Opportunity for service and education abroad
- ❑ Increased industrialization
- ❑ The nursing students has got a status of a student
- ❑ Extension of community health services
- ❑ Government support to health programs
- ❑ Increased number of private nursing homes
- ❑ Development of nursing research
- ❑ Changing role of women in society
- ❑ Empowerment of women
- ❑ Computerization of medical services.

For all above reasons the carrier opportunities are increasing day-by-day. The choice of field for practice depends upon interest, qualification, availability of opportunity.

Hospital Nursing Services

Mainly nursing revolves around the hospitals and clinical areas. Thus the nurse in the hospital will be actively involved in many different ways in meeting comprehensive needs of patients, i.e. physical, emotional, spiritual and social needs.

Possible positions available for the nurses in the hospital are:

- ■ Staff nurse (minimum qualification should be GNM)
- ■ Ward sister
- ■ Departmental supervisor
- ■ Assistant nursing superintendent (ANS)
- ■ Deputy nursing superintendent (DNS)
- ■ Nursing superintendent (NS)
- ■ Chief nursing officer (CNO)
- ■ Director of nursing at state level health services
- ■ In-service education director
- ■ Clinical nurse specialist in various medical specialties
- ■ Nurse researcher
- ■ Private duty nurse
- ■ Home sister or warden

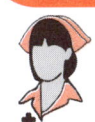

If the hospital is a teaching institution for nurses, she will also be involved in clinical supervision of the nursing students and participating in ward teaching program for students and staff.

Nurse also got opportunity in the nursing educational institutes. Mainly two types of educational institutes are present.

1. **School of nursing:** Where ANM and GNM diploma is awarded.
2. **College of nursing**: These are for the graduation degree, postgraduation degrees and PhD programs.

Careers available in school/college of nursing are as follow:

In School of Nursing

- Sister tutor
- Clinical instructor or clinical supervisor
- Principal tutor
- Public health nurse or community health nurse.

In College of Nursing

- Junior lecturer
- Senior lecturer
- Reader
- Associate professor
- Professor
- Principal
- Director
- Assistant director of public health nursing.

Community Health Nursing

Earlier known as public health nursing is now community health nursing. In 1951 Bhore report recommendations gives a boost to community health nursing. Opening of primary health care centers, dispensaries, subcenters, rural health care centers gives more opportunities to the nursing field. Advanced study in public health nursing is greatly encouraged by the government.

The career opportunities available in this area are:

- Community health nurse at PHC, CHC
- Nurse in school health program
- District public health nursing officer
- Community health nursing teacher

Industrial Nursing

With the implementation of Factory Act of 1948 all large industries to employ the medical officer and nurses in the factory for the health and medical well-being of their employees. The specialization in industrial nursing in now available after the degree program. Most of the time she is responsible for the prevention of accidents and industrial hazards.

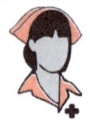

Military Nursing

The military nursing services is a part of Indian army. Nurses become commissioned officer and are given rank from lieutenant to a brigadier. The main responsibility of the military nurse is at the time of war and peace. She has to serve in military hospitals as well as at any area of the country at time of need. The nurse in army service must have a real sense of courage, sense of duty and devotion.

Private Duty Nurse

It is not very common practice due to high cost and high family values in India but very much practiced in abroad. Nowadays many private nursing bureaus have come up.

Nursing Services Abroad

Nursing services in abroad is a very attractive choice of the nurses. Good salaries, facilities and professional growth opportunities are the major attractions. A number of companies and institutes provide the facilities for nursing services in aboard. The nursing exchange program by the universities is also one opportunity.

Nursing Services in Other Areas

- Nurses registrar at state level
- Trained nurses association secretary
- Indian nursing council secretary
- Nursing advisor to government of India at national level
- Red cross nursing services
- Research and writing and editing jobs
- Dean for nursing services in different universities.

Choosing wisely from the varied opportunity developed for nurses is a difficult task. Before choosing the career one should assess and evaluate one's ability and capability. Whatever a nurse chooses should be done with great responsibility.

IN-SERVICE EDUCATION

In-service education as name indicates refers to an ongoing-on-the-job instruction that is given to enhance, the worker's performance in their present job.

Definition

- In-service education is a planned learning experience provided by the employing agency for employees.
- In-service education is a planned educational experience provided in the job setting and closely identified with service in order to help the person to perform more effectively as a person and as a worker (NLN).
- In-service education is defined as a continued program of education provided by the employing authority, with the purpose of developing the competence of personnel in their functions appropriate to the position they hold or to which they will be appointed in the services.

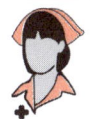

Aims

- To keep improvement of performance
- Acquisition of new knowledge
- To keep in face in changing society to their needs
- Improvement of client through upgrading the services rendered with scientific principles
- To develop specific skills required for practice, improves the staff members chances for promotion
- To develop right concept of patients care and maintain the high standards of nursing
- At work situation in-service education reduces mechanical action to a minimum and promotes economy, safety and office of the person
- It helps in the reduction of turnover and absenteeism.

Components

The main components of in-service education are as follow:
- Orientation skills training program
- Continuing education program
- Leadership training and management skills development
- Staff development program

To be successful in conducting such program, the hospital administration staff must believe firmly the value of in-service education as a tool to improve performance and attitudes of staff and is absolutely essential.

Orientation Skill Training Program

Orientation skill training program introduces a new employee to these basic aspects of her job. In the hospital/clinical field when new nurse is appointed. The supervisor has to discuss with them about job chart, policies of the area, objectives, procedures, standing orders, work situations, etc. so that she may easily got adjustment in the area and new environment and can do the work efficiently.

So orientation skill training has to be given for development of knowledge and skills.

Continuing Education

Rapid scientific progress is an important reason for continued education program. The changes in medical sciences and other sciences are taking place at tremendous rate. Everyday some new knowledge, new discoveries are added. Inventions in many branches of science make changes in medical and nursing practice necessary. These changes are so rapid that it is difficult to keep pace with it unless there is a definite organized plan to conduct continued education programs.

Types are as follows:
- **Centralized in-service training:** One department will be there which will held the response for the improvement of knowledge, skills, practice of their nursing staff.
- **Decentralized in-service educations:** This is planned for the staff members who work together and program are planned around the special relevant interest of the employees.
- **Combined or coordinated in-service education approach:** There will be a central nursing in-service education department consists of nurses in each division, who holds leadership responsibility for staff development activities, whose time is devoted fully for teaching, learning experience and situation. They plan, conduct, evaluate the program and further plan their program based on the need arises.

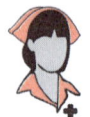

❑ **Management skills and leadership training:** Mainly this type of in-service education is imparted to the administrators and the senior personnels. This is for the persons possess high qualifications and who is having the chances of promotion or supervisors. Through in-service education managerial skills, supervising tacts and leadership qualities are imparted to achieve the targets by reaching goals and preparing the persons to solve their problems if any need arises and to have smooth environment in their working areas.

❑ **Staff development program:** To meet the educational and managerial needs of nursing students and staff, there must be provision for regular staff development program which should have the following main components:
- Orientation
- In-service education
- Self-instructions and continuing education
- Attending short-term courses, workshops, seminars, presentations, etc.

Value of In-service Education

In-service education program is basically to improve the performance and attitudes of staff with the upcoming challenges in nursing, emerging from the phenomena of change about the functions in health and illness, the professionals roles are altered. To meet this altered changes of development in-service education have a great role of play.

It helps the professionals to recognize the current social changes and future ones for seen, and prepare themself for these changes.

Everyday new researches, new models, new theories emerge in nursing. To centralize all these thing in-service education program are there.

In nutshell as part of staff development program, it includes various areas or components like orientation, skill training, technical training, leadership, management training, safety training and various other essential aspects.

Need Participation in Committee Procedure

Committee is the group of experts who plans and reaches to some conclusion or decision is taken. Or

Committees are the vehicles through which the educational enterprise in managed usually consists of one overriding committee or bound with various subcommittees.

The committees have seven or more members including both senses, representatives of general educational and health interests of community with hospital administrator, nursing institutional administrator serving as ex-office members.

There are a number of types of committees. These can be classified as:
- Based on tenure
- Based on structure

Base on Tenure

❑ Temporary committees
❑ Permanent committees

Based on Structure

❑ Formal
❑ Informal

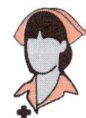

Committees can be setup at all two levels:
- An advisory committee (At the level of controlling body)
- Standing committee (For among the school or college staff)

The main functions of these committees are:
- Informing itself regarding nursing education and studying the needs of educational institutes.
- Nominating to the board of trustees, the director of the institute, and approving, upon his/her nomination and all other faculty members.
- Passing upon policies recommended by the faculty of the institute and supporting the faculty in maintaining these policies
- Seeing that the requisite teaching staff is available
- Delegating authority to the director of the institute
- Approving the budget for recommendation to the controlling body.
- Concerning itself with the general welfare and social life of students
- Assisting in interpreting the aims of institute to the public
- Safeguarding the interest of the institute in all ways.

As these all committees are working for the welfare of the profession so it is necessary to participate in committee procedures.

NURSING IN FUTURE

Nursing is the oldest of arts and youngest of professions. It is the integral part of the health care system, encompasses the promotion of health, prevention of illness and rehabilitative services.

Nursing is not an easy job. It continue to be challenged and rewarded with the opportunities and constraints. In the future the nursing have to face the challenges grab the opportunities and meet the changes in a positive way. A number of significant issues are there which affect the development of the profession like:
- Professional and self-image of nurses
- Societal images and expectations of nurses
- Degree of nursing profession control over the quality and quantity of practitioners
- Impact of technology and theory on nursing practices roles and settings
- Sources of financing for health care service.

As prediction of the future nursing is an occupation fraught with peril in a society and world changing rapidly. The changes will be accomplished by changes in both nursing practice and nursing education.

Nursing research is one which brings the future nursing to a top level. Use of computers, use of number of technical tools help to meet the new challenges of the future nursing. As the change in nursing education and nursing practice is there, that signs toward the bright future of the nursing practices.

ASSESS YOURSELF

1. Define continue education? Give meaning, importance, scope, need and opportunities of continuing education.
2. What is in-service education? Plan an in-service education program for ANM's of your area.
3. Write the scope of nursing career.

15 Legislation in Nursing

Learning Objectives

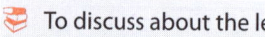 To discuss about the legal aspects of nursing.

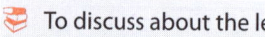 To describe the rules, regulations to save nurses and patients rights.

Key Terms

- **Legislation:** Law which has been promulgated by a governing body.
- **Disaster:** A sudden accident or natural catastrophe that causes great damage or loss of life.
- **Crime:** Forbidden act punishable by law.
- **License:** A permission (in written form) given by any authentic authority to do a specific thing.

Legal responsibility in nursing practice is becoming of greater importance as each year passes. The main aim of studying this chapter or knowing the legislation in nursing is:

- To better understand your legal responsibilities in nursing practice
- To recognize by what authorities those responsibilities can be enforced
- To become more aware and alert to the areas of nursing practice in which legal difficulties are most likely to arise.

PURPOSE AND IMPORTANCE OF LAWS IN NURSING

The main purpose of knowing the laws in nursing are as follows:

- This helps the nurse to protect herself from legal involvement
- The knowledge of law protects the rights of clients and nurses
- She should know by what authority these laws can be enforced.

IMPORTANCE OR VALUE OF LAWS IN NURSING

- The knowledge of law has great value in nursing as it differentiates the nursing practice from the practice of other health care professionals. It describes and protects the rights of patients as well as the nurses. It protects the patients against deliberate injury by a nurse. These laws

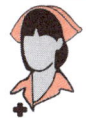

specify the nurse's responsibilities towards patients; regulate a nurse's relationship with doctors. The main importance is that it specify the nurse's duty to protect public and her duty for record keeping and records.

There are many instances when the nurses have to abide by the law. Some of them are as follows:

❑ A patient who comes to the hospital has all the rights as a citizen and his entry denotes his willingness to undergo any investigation or treatment or an operation in which anesthetic is used, requires the written consent of the patient. If the patient is above the age of 18 years and has sound state of mind, consent should be taken by him/her if he/she is less than 18 years the consent from parents or guardian should be taken. If any problem occurs, senior ward sister, surgeon and the administrative officer can be informed.

❑ The nurse and midwife has a serious responsibility in making sure that all the babies born in the hospital are correctly labeled at birth by giving them identity bands so that at no time they can be placed in the wrong bed or given away to the wrong mother. Greater care is necessary when dealing with young children or unconscious patients to ensure correct identity.

In the operation theater the scrubbed nurse must check the number of all the instruments, needle, sponges and check all items used. She should make a final check-up before the cavity is closed.

There are two acts which control the use of drugs in treatment. They are:

1. Poisonous Drug Act.

2. Food and Drug Act: The prescriptions should note:
   ▪ The name and address of the patient
   ▪ The date
   ▪ Signature of prescriber
   ▪ Total quantity to be supplied in words or figures.

In hospitals the use of poisonous drugs is under strict control. Each hospital has a protocol to have and maintain the accurate record of each poisonous drug.

❑ Accidents may occur to the patients or visitors or employees of the hospital due to negligence. Hospital staff should be aware of their responsibilities and be alert to the risks entailed being them to notice of the concerned authorities. Any member of the staff who has been negligent or incompetent and has caused injury to a patient may be found guilty of culpable negligence and damages will be awarded against her personally.

❑ Sometimes the patient may demand that he may be discharged though the medical advice, it is against nursing ethics. It is the duty of the nurse to persuade him not to do so. But if the patient insisted that he should be discharged, the nurse should inform the doctor. If the patient does not even listen to doctors, advice he should be asked to give in writing a statement to the effect that he is taking discharge on his own responsibility and risk. If he does not agree to it even then a note to this effect should be made and signed by two witness.

❑ All hospitals have a protocol to tell that hospital cannot take responsibility of valuables and money. Care should be taken to see that instead of gold, silver or platinum, yellow metal or white metal should be written.

❑ In most hospitals there is a rule against the nurse signing the legal documents or witnessing signatures during their professional duties.

❑ The nurse should report immediately to the authorities concerned whenever any theft has occurred in the hospital.

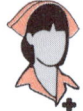

❑ Professional secrecy is another important law. Whatever confidential information given by the patient, should not be revealed to any one even though they may be his close relatives. The details of the patient's disease should not be informed to the employer as it may cause loss to the patient by way of removal from service for which the nurse may be legally hold responsible. Discretion must be used by the nurses in giving information about the patient's progress.

CENTRAL AND STATE LEGISLATIONS

Six kinds of authorities used as guides to legal responsibility of the nurse are:
❑ Central and State Government Acts
❑ The International Code for Nurses
❑ Institutional Rules and Regulations
❑ Standing Orders
❑ Precedent

The central government is a source of legal authority in three ways. They are:
1. Government Service Conduct Rules
2. The Indian Nursing Council Act
3. Law Based upon the English Pattern

Government Service Conduct Rule

There are detailed rules of conduct for all government employees. Requirement to maintain absolute integrity, devotion to duty, and high standard of moral behavior are some of the examples of these rules. Some of these are applicable to nursing practice. All these rules are applicable to the government employees. These conduct rules may be used as a basis for developing specific rules for the nursing practice.

Indian Nursing Council Act

This is the main and only legislation which is directly related to nursing practice. It is a basis from which rules for nursing practice can be developed. The Indian Nursing Council Act gives authority to the Indian Nursing Council, among other responsibilities, for prescribing curricula for nursing education and recognizing qualifications of institutions with teaching program. The INC uses this authority in nursing education but it delegates authority for control of nursing practice to the state nurses registration councils.

Law Based upon the English Pattern

It is the third way in which the central government is a source of legal authority. These laws are very specific and make the nurse, "liable for negligence" or answerable to the law for acts of carelessness.

A brief summary of the laws are given below which are applicable for all medical practitioners including nursing:

❑ **Right to refuse to treat a patient** except in an emergency situation. Though it is doubtful that a patient would be refused treatment, it is supported by law.

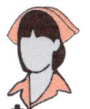

- **Right to sue for fees:** This is applicable only to private duty nurses or private practitioners. The other nurses get salaries and so, such situations do not occur. The right to add a tittle or description to one's name. The nurse may add any title, description abbreviation or letter implying the holding a degree, diploma, license or certificate showing particular qualifications may be added. Its improper use is prohibited by State Nurses Registration Acts. The right to wear the red cross emblem is given only to the members of army medical services.

- Unregistered practitioners are not allowed to hold positions or appointments in public and local hospitals.

- There are certain fundamental duties for the nurse. They are:
    - The nurse should exercise a seasonable degree of skill and knowledge in treating patients.
    - Once the patient comes in contact with the nurse it is her obligation to attend the patient as long as necessary unless the patient wish to withdraw or notice is given to his intention to withdraw.
    - A nurse who is practicing must give personal attention to her cases and answer calls promptly.
    - Care should be taken to children from harming themselves.
    - Special care must be taken in the case of adults who are incapable of taking care of themselves.
    - The Indian Penal Code demands that poisonous drugs should be kept in separate containers properly labeled and marked. They should not be mixed with nonpoisonous drugs.
    - The nurse has a duty to secrecy to the patients. Records should be kept confidential. The practitioner may reveal the content only when called upon to give evidence in court.
    - Dangerous diseases must be reported.
    - Nurses are considered solely responsible for their professional acts whoever be the employing authority.

    The state government has control over nursing practice through the State Nurses Registration Acts.

SERVICE CONDUCT AND INSTITUTIONAL LAWS

The state nurse's registration councils have authority to prescribe rules of conduct. They can take disciplinary action and they maintain registers of nurses, midwifes and others. Most states have Acts that prevent registration or remove from the register. Removal from the register may be due to the following offences:

- Conviction for a nonbailable offence
- If found guilty of conduct indicating that the individual is unfit for registration
- If she possesses defects in character

The state has prohibited the following unethical practices:

- The dishonest use of certificates
- Procuring registration by false means
- Falsification of register
- Representation of registration by an unrecognized person.

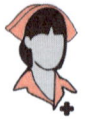

COMMON LEGAL HAZARDS IN NURSING

There are certain areas in nursing practice which have legal implications. Prevention of any possibility to harm the patient from the environment or from his care is the duty of a nurse.

There may be many hazards in the environment such as slippery floors, faulty equipment, absence of railing on stairways, presence of inflammable substance, inadequate protection from stray animals, inadequate lighting, absence of bedside rails and electrical wiring, etc.

Procedures in nursing needs special attention and care because of legal implications are:

- Having written orders from the physician for treatment and care of the patient
- To register births, deaths, still birth and all vital statistics
- Administering medicines, giving only as ordered checking labels and appearances of medicines, charting accurately
- To administer cold or hot applications to the body especially for patients unable to respond cannot tell the nurse when they are having pain or harmful reactions
- Getting permission slips signed for surgery or other treatment (consents)
- Identifying patients including babies and identifying bodies
- To report accidents, errors and incompetent behavior

Negligence or carelessness in all the above areas can bring about serious legal difficulties particularly as patients become more aware of their right to a certain quality of care. The nurse can protect herself and the patient best by being aware of legal implications and by maintaining a high standard of nursing. The institution where the nursing student is studying or where the nurse is working assumes the protection of the nursing student or nurse.

The Trained Nurses Association of India (TNAI) may also provide some legal aid to its members when required.

DISASTER (EMERGENCY) SITUATIONS

In an ordinary emergency situation, the nurse should give necessary treatment to preserve life until the arrival of a physician. When an emergency involves many people, such as war, flood, and accidents etc. the usual restriction on the activities and responsibilities of the nurse are removed. In the absence of medical practitioner or personnel, the nurse has to take the responsibilities, ordinarily carried by the doctor. The nurse may have to diagnose and treat patients and do many procedures usually prohibited by law for nursing practice. In the emergency or disaster situations mentioned above, the nurse has to treat the patients irrespective of their nationality, whether they are the enemies, civilians or military. No favoritism should be shown in giving priority in the order of treatment. It is the main duty of the nurse to do everything possible to care for the wounded and sick, protect them from harm and violence and also prevent the spread of infections. If the nurse practices in this way she will be legally protected by both the Red Cross Principles and the International Code for Nurses. So it is important that the nurses should be well aware of what they may or may not do according to Geneva Convention of 1949. These conventions are universally recognized. They are supported by most countries throughout the world. The Red Cross principles under the conventions very clearly states the "Rights and Duties of Nurses" in the document published in 1973. Legal protection will always be available for the nurse if she practices according to the principles stated above. She will be protected by both Red Cross Principles and Intervention Code for Nurses. At the same time, she is expected to give the highest standard of nursing care possible under the circumstances.

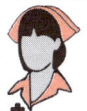

LEGISLATION IN NURSING

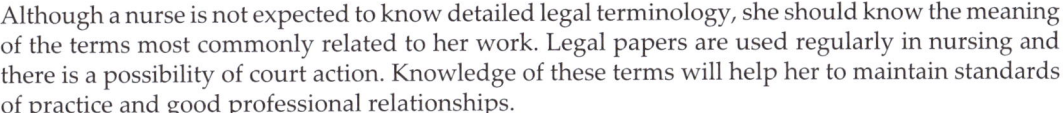

Legal Terms

Although a nurse is not expected to know detailed legal terminology, she should know the meaning of the terms most commonly related to her work. Legal papers are used regularly in nursing and there is a possibility of court action. Knowledge of these terms will help her to maintain standards of practice and good professional relationships.

- **An Act:** It is the written law, which has been formally passed by the government
- **The Bill:** It is a draft or temporary outline of what the act will be
- **Legal document:** Document accurately written which is signed and dated by the person who prepared it and has legal value.
- **Agreement bond:** A signing contract of conditions.
- **License:** A written permission given by a recognized authority to do a specific thing.
- **Will:** A written statement of a person, what he wants to do with his property after his death.
- **Witness:** A person who under oath gives testimony in court to help to decide case.
- **Summons:** Written notice calling a person to appear in court.
- **Crime:** A forbidden act punishable by law.
- **Narcotic law:** A specific law which controls the purchasing and giving out of narcotic drugs.

Regulations of Nursing Education

The several studies conducted on nursing education suggested and consistently made five recommendations which becomes the regulations of nursing education.

- The nursing education programs should be established within the system of higher education.
- Nurses should be highly educated.
- The student nurses should not be used to staff hospitals.
- The standards exist for nursing practice.
- All nurses should have a minimum qualification of graduation, on the basis of that the following nursing programs are established:
    - **ANM:** Auxiliary nurse midwives training program for 2 years.
    - **GNM:** General nurse and midwifery training program for 3 years.
    - **Post certificate BSc:** Nursing degree program for 2 years.

Registration and Reciprocities

A registration is very important for every nurse to practice nursing legally. Every nurse who completes the degree or diploma course according to the syllabus of INC through a recognized institute can get the registration in the State Nursing Council. Registration system helps to maintain the high standard of nursing care and profession.

Registration gives legal protection to the nurse and also to the public by preventing unqualified and incompetent people to practice nursing.

Institute and the student nurse have to file online online-application for the registration in State Council with supporting documents. Then the Registration Council registers their names and issue them the registration number.

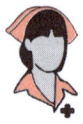

Renewal or reciprocities of the registration of the person is done to keep control on practicing the profession in state. The process to get the renewal certificate is almost same as registration. A renewal certificate is issued to the person by the State Council.

The registration certificate serves as a legal pool of registry and renewal certificate indicates that she is still in active practice. Therefore this must be preserved by every nurse for future practice.

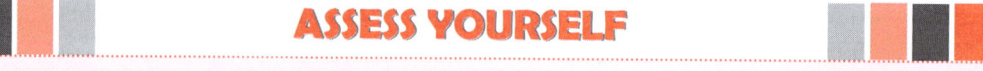

ASSESS YOURSELF

1. Do you think legislation in nursing is must. Give comments.
2. What are the common legal hazards in nursing?
3. Give details for the legal responsibilities of a professional nurse.

Professional and Related Organizations

16

Learning Objectives

- Students will learn about the professional and related organizations.
- To discuss about the role of professional organizations in human kind and health matters.

Key Terms

- **Esprit de corps:** Union is strength or unity.
- **Professional organizations:** Organizations to strengthen the profession. These are backbone of profession.
- **TNAI:** Trained Nurses Association of India.

PROFESSIONAL ORGANIZATIONS

In every profession there are professional organizations. These organizations are the backbone of the profession, so one must be aware of the professional organizations of his/her own profession. As a nurse, we must know what different professional organizations/bodies are there in the country and abroad so that we can participate in all activities and development of the profession. Professional organizations provide the opportunities to express the view points and help to develop the leadership abilities by keeping all the news and trends at your door step.

Registration is extremely important for you to become a licensed professional nurse. As it is the document which allows you to function officially as professional nurse.

TRAINED NURSES ASSOCIATION OF INDIA (TNAI)

The TNAI stands for Trained Nurses Association of India. It is the national professional association of nurses. In 1905 in Lucknow Miss Allen Martin as president and Miss Burn as secretary formed association of nursing superintendents and named it 'Association of Nursing Superintendents'. Then in 1908 at Bombay, a decision was made to establish a trained nurses association and accordingly the association was inaugurated in 1909. Later on in 1922 both organizations came together and merged. It was decided to establish only one organization that was TNAI (Trained Nurses Association of India).

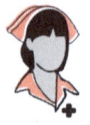

In 1905 nine European nurses were holding the administrative posts in India and laid objectives:
- Upholding the dignity and honor of the nursing profession
- Promoting a sense of esprit de corps among all nurses
- Enabling members to take counsel together on matters related to their profession.

The organization of TNAI makes it possible for all nurses to participate at all levels beginning with the local units. The level of organization moves for city branches to district level, state and national level. Members of TNAI are most active at city and state level branches. Some state level branches of TNAI have full time secretaries. Active members can participate on the state level through service on executive committee of the state branch. This group of active member is called 'INTEREST GROUP'. It concentrates its activities on a specific area of practice in nursing. Nursing education, nursing administration, community health nursing and psychiatry nursing are some of the specific area.

The governing body of the TNAI is council. This is assisted by standing committees for economy welfare, nursing research and finance. A full time secretary was appointed in 1935. A salaried assistant secretary was also appointed. He serves as the advisor to SNA. He was appointed in 1983.

The aim of the TNAI center upon needs of the individual member and the problems in the nursing profession as whole. The aims are as follows:
- Upgrading, development and standardization of nursing education and elevating nursing education
- Improvement of living and working conditions for nurses and educational conditions for nurses and to elevate economic welfare of nurse in country. In every state TNAI has directed the state government to appoint a nurse as a nursing director
- Registration for qualified nurse and reciprocity of registration within different states in the country as well as within different countries.

Membership in the TNAI is obtained by application with a copy of her state registration certificate. Membership from the student nurse association is given after sanding a certificate from the institution where she studied within 6 months after completing the course. Membership fee is charged for membership of the TNAI, but a reduced fee is offered to those who transfer membership from student nurses association. Part of these fees is used for affiliation to the International Council of Nurses, TNAI offers life membership also. Membership of TNAI is a practice for employment in many institutions.

The official organ of TNAI is 'The Nursing Journal of India' which is published monthly. The cost of this journal is included in the annual subscription for membership of TNAI. Indian nursing year book is another impressive publication of TNAI. It has been published five times since 1982. It contains important reports, discussions of trends and statistics required by the nursing profession in India. Its list of 'who is who' has grown with each publication.

The policy of TNAI is to work with the government and other authorities and guard against the tendency of adopting unethical and unprofessional means to mitigate grievances.

The TNAI took the initiative to celebrate the health related days like WHO day, international nurses day and nurses week. It gives an opportunity for the get together to nurses and discuss matters pertaining to health and nursing. TNAI incorporates health visitors leagues, midwives and auxiliary nurse midwives association and students nurses association in 1929. It is associated with many national and international associations such as International Council of Nurses, National Council of Women in India, Tuberculosis Association of India, etc.

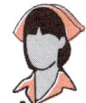

The students can get their registration in TNAI after the completion of their basic course which they are doing with a certificate from the institute.

A professional nurse in also benefitted from membership of TNAI (Fig. 1). It gives the feeling of belonging and security because the numbers of nurses are united through the organization. Professional activities give ample opportunity to develop leadership ability and professional poise, keep abreast of changes, and share and solve the professional problems. The journals help to obtain the information about the current affairs in nursing and, offer opportunities to publish articles and voice one's opinions. TNAI can help to apply for career position, if desired. It helps economically by providing scholarships for advanced study, railway concessions for nursing students and staff nurses and limited income for welfare aid when necessary.

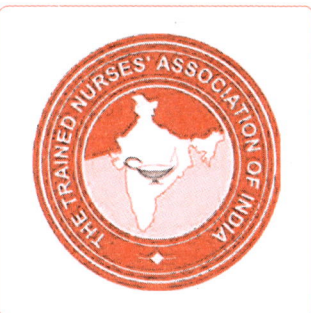

Fig. 1: Emblem of TNAI

STUDENT NURSES ASSOCIATION (SNA)

The SNA was organized in 1920. It is associated with and works under the jurisdiction of TNAI. It provides a means of personal professional development for nursing students. It serves as source of membership for TNAI. The assistant secretary of TNAI serves as the advisor to SNA The membership of the TNAI gives them a sense of security and belonging keeps them in touch with the latest changes in nursing. It helps them to share and solve personal problems and development of leadership qualities.

The objectives of the SNA are:

- To help students to uphold the dignity and ideals of the profession for which they are qualifying.
- To promote a corporate spirit among students for the common good cause.
- To furnish nurses in training within their courses of study leading to professional qualifications.
- To encourage leadership ability and help students to gain a wide knowledge of the nursing profession in all its different branches and aspects.
- To increase the student nurses social contacts and general knowledge in order to help them with their total personal and professional development.
- To encourage both professional and recreational meetings games and sports.
- To provide a special section in the Nursing Journal of India for the benefit of students.
- To encourage students to compete for prizes in the students nurses exhibition and to attend national and regional conferences. The whole organization of SNA is similar to that of TNAI. Local units are established in the institutions. The diary of various events is kept by SNA secretary. The diaries from all the entire unit are presented at the time of national conferences. The SNA unit later on moves to national levels as TNAI.
- With the help of student nurses develop a cooperative spirit with other student nurses which will help them in future professional relationship.
- To provide a means of having a voice in what the association stands for and does.

Organization of activities in the SNA is similar to that of the TNAI. The first level of organ is the local unit established in a teaching institution. Then there are the state and national levels just in the TNAI. The local unit has a unit executive committee consists of a president acts as SNA advisor and the remaining officers are students. The president is a professional nurse. She is a member of

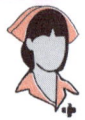

the TNAI serves only as an advisor. The vice president and the secretary are the students. State level advisors are active members of the TNAI elected by the state branches. There is a full time secretary on the national level at the national headquarters located in New Delhi. She is a member of TNAI appointed by the TNAI council and part of the national level SNA general committee.

Membership fees in SNA are normal and easily met by the nursing students. It is possible to transfer membership to TNAI conveniently. TNAI makes such arrangements. Nursing students participating in the student nurses association have an excellent opportunity to development leadership abilities, social poise and competitive skills and an interest in the profession as a whole. The association and its relationship with the TNAI is also helpful to the nursing students in many ways. Problems in nursing education and problems related to the living conditions of the nurses can be solved through the joint afford of TNAI and SNA.

INTERNATIONAL COUNCIL OF NURSES (ICN)

The ICN (Fig. 2), founded in 1899 by Mrs Bedford Fenwick. It is a federation of a nonpolitical and self-governing National Nurses Association. The headquarters is in Geneva, Switzerland. The main purpose of this council is to provide an opportunity to share the interests in the promotion of health and care of the sick the national councils. Great emphasis is paid on nondiscrimination ICN accepts into membership of one association of nurses per country. There are 15 countries National Organization which are members of this council.

Its main objectives are:

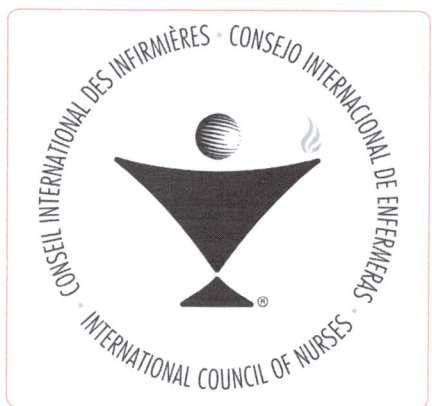

Fig. 2: Emblem of ICN

❑ To promote the development of strong national nurses association.

❑ To assist national nurse associations to improve the standard of nursing and competences of nurses.

❑ To assist national nurses associations to improve the status of nurses within their countries.

❑ To serve as the authoritative voice for nurses and nursing internationals.

The international council is the global voice of nursing. It is one of the activities and accomplishment is the publication of the code for nurses. The worldwide accepted definition of a nurse and the nurses dilemma, a book of ethics are given by ICN. It makes policy statements on health and social issues and offers a great variety of seminars and statements for maintaining and improving the status of the nurse and the standard of nursing in the world. The guidelines for National Nurses Associations in the Indian nursing year book 1988–89, is an example of how the council works for the improvement of nursing education and practice.

The governing body of the ICN is the council of national representatives which is made up of the ICN honorary officers and the president of the national member associations. The council meets on alternate years and once every 4 years at the time of ICN congress. At the headquarters work is carried out by a staff of clerical and expert nursing advisory personnel. ICN publishes the international nursing review on a quarterly basis. The newsletter published 10 times a year gives news of the ICN activities and the national member associations. All nurses can become members of the ICN not individually but only if his/her national nurses association is a member of

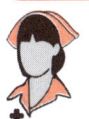

the ICN. Nurses in India become the member of ICN if they are members of TNAI. Affiliation for this membership is paid from a portion of the member fees paid to the TNAI.

Membership of ICN through TNAI has various benefits to her as an individual nurse. A limited number of nursing students may have their expenses paid to attend conferences and congresses as observers. The graduate nurse gets several benefits like attendance of international congresses or conferences. The exchange of privileges program, professional advice or assistance through ICN headquarters and by using the ICN information center. The nurses who are members of ICN can get publications about development of nursing and nursing education around the world. It helps nurse to become aware of being professionally related to international organizations such as United Nations and WHO.

INDIAN NURSING COUNCIL (INC)

The INC, which was authorized by the Indian Nursing Council Act of 1947, was established in 1949 for the purpose of providing uniform standards in nursing education and reciprocity in nursing registration throughout the country. Nurses registered in one state were not necessarily recognized for registration in another state before this time. The condition of mutual recognition by the state nurse's registration councils, which is called reciprocity, was possible only if uniform standards of nursing education were maintained. Therefore the INC was given authority to prescribe curricula for nursing education in all the states. It was also given authority to recognize program of nursing education or to refuse recognition of a program if it did not meet the standards required by the council.

Additional responsibilities were given to the INC when the initial Indian Nursing Council Act of 1947 was amended in 1957. The INC was then asked to provide for registration of foreign nurses and for the maintenance of the Indian nurses register. This register contains the names of all nurses, midwives, auxiliary nurse midwives and 'para-nursing' workers who are enrolled on all state register.

The INC authorized State Nurses Registration Councils and Examining Boards to issue qualifying certificates. This recognition is given, however only after those bodies have been recognized by their state government.

The INC has been given heavy responsibilities for nursing practice and nursing education. It has not been able to exert enough power to supply high standards in nursing as some private diploma and degree program which have no approval of INC or State Council are growing in number, same time some untrained and unlicensed nursing personnel used to staff these institutions.

The Indian Nursing Council is composed the representative of state registration council, central and state health departments, military nursing services, Indian Red Cross Society, university school of nursing health schools and post certificate schools TNAI, Medical Council of India, Indian Medical Association and three Members of Parliament. The INC maintains a register of all nurses in country.

STATE NURSING COUNCIL AND REGISTRATION

Registration in State Nursing Council is very necessary for every nurse. It is necessary to be registered in order to function officially as a professional nurse. Registration councils are functioning in all the states of India and they are affiliated to INC.

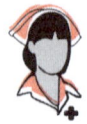

A register of names of professional nurses is maintained by each state nurse's registration council. These names are also put into the Indian nurses register maintained by the Indian nursing council nurses, midwives, auxiliary nurse midwives and health visitors are registered. All degree holding nurses also have to get the registration in State Council.

The present function of state nurses registration council are:

- State council is accredited body. It recognize officially and inspect schools of nursing in their state
- State council conduct examination
- Prescribe rules of conduct, take disciplinary actions etc.
- Maintain registers of graduate nurses, nurses holding degrees in nursing, auxiliary nurse midwives, or multipurpose workers and health visitors.

The State Nursing Council is independent and recognized as a body who can make status and prescribed by laws for trained nurses and nurses who are undergoing various courses of studies. Although it works independent, it has to obtain approval from state government for the by-laws passed by it and decisions taken.

Punjab Nurses Registration Council is in Chandigarh and is commonly known as PNRC. It is administratively headed by the registrar who usually is a nurse. The deputy registrar is also a nurse. There is other staff like accountants, LDCs, UDCs, peons, drivers, etc. who the registrar in her day-to-day work and functions. The main functions of registrar in PNRC are:

- To arrange for inspections to ascertain that institutes are carrying out educational program as per syllabus, conditions and rules and regulation
- Helps and inspect the criteria's to open a new school of nursing
- To draw a program for examination of various types of educational program at all centers at same time
- To prepare a time schedule for written and practical examinations to prepare roll number sheets of students and send them to various examination centers
- To get question papers etc. printed under strict confidential atmosphere and keep up secrecy regarding them
- To prepare examination results and communicate the same to all concerned institutions
- To prepare diploma certificates, registration certificates of nurses who have successfully qualified for both
- To help the State Council to take action against the persons whose written reports are received for not abiding by the regulations of Punjab Nursing Council either at the time of examinations or in nursing practice as a professional nurse.

Registration

All the nurses who have undergone any diploma, degree course and certificate course should register themself in the State Nursing Council.

Registration is an important task for professionals as it serves as legal protection to the nurse and also to public as it prevents unqualified and in complex persons practicing nursing.

The State Nursing Council can expert official control of standards of nursing practice through Registrar system.

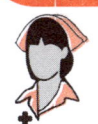

Registration Procedure

The institution where the student has received education usually initiates the registration process. The examining authority usually the State Nursing Council issues a diploma to nurse after she successfully completes the recognized educational program. She should apply to the registration council for a form which has to be properly filled by her and along with the certificate from hospital authority stating the she has completed the course, is sent to registrar along with the required fees. The Xerox copy of the diploma certificate also has to be attached to the form while applying for registration in midwifery.

After going through all the details in the form and attached documents the name of the nurse in entered in state register maintained in council and registration certificate is issued to the person, which bears the registration number and the part of the register in which the name is registered.

COMMONWEALTH NURSES FEDERATION (CNF)

The TNAI is also affiliated with the commonwealth nurses federation which is a nurse association begun by the commonwealth foundation. It is made up of nurses associations from commonwealth countries. The headquarters of the federation is in London.

The aim of this organization is, in general to promote sharing, better communications and closer relationships between its member associations. It also provides expert professional advice, scholarships for advanced study, financial assistance for professional meetings and seminars and an office through which funds can be received and disbursed for benefit of nursing in the countries which are represented.

The commonwealth nurses, federation was formally organized in 1973 and operates in six regions of world which are East, Central and Southern Africa, Africa West Atlantic, Australia, Far east and Pacific, South Asia and Europe. Beginning with 25 member countries it is now represented in 62 independent nations.

NURSES LEAGUE OF THE CHRISTIAN MEDICAL ASSOCIATION

The nurses league of the Christian Medical Association of India was founded in 1930 as the nurses auxiliary of CMAI. The name was changed from nurse auxiliary to nurses, league in 1965. It became affiliated to the TNAI in 1936 and promotes membership in this organization.

The nurses league of the CMAI was originally organized to meet the needs felt by Christian nurses to share common problems related to training and registration of nurses.

The current objectives are to:

❑ Promote cooperation and encouragement among Christian nurses

❑ Promote efficiency in nursing education and service, encourage the highest quality of candidates to choose nursing as vocation

❑ Secure the highest standards possible in Christian nursing education through the Christian school nursing

❑ Consider the special work and problems of Christian nurses wherever employed specially in isolated areas.

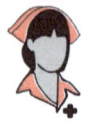

The nurses league has a full time secretary. Until 1986 it published *The Christian Nurse* bimonthly but now limits regular publications to a column in CMAI newsletter. Membership fees are required and a life membership is available. Nursing students may become associate member of the league. Membership in the nursing league, may be a requirement for certain positions under control of Christian employing authorities.

Special activities of nurses' league included national and area conferences and retreats for its membership. Development of leadership abilities is encouraged by participation these meetings where professional papers and exhibits of high quality are given.

The nurses league has two examination boards which are recognized by the INC one is the *Mid-India Board of Examinees* and other is the *Board of Nursing Education* in south India. These bodies direct examinations in GNM and diplomas granted by them are accepted for registration with states in those areas. Another major contribution of these boards has been and continues to be the overseeing of the preparation of textbooks and manuals for nursing education in India. Participation in professional organizations is of profit to the nurse and profession. The profession provides a means through which united efforts can be made to improve standards of nursing education and practice.

RELATED ORGANIZATIONS AND THEIR CONTRIBUTION TO NURSING

World Health Organization (WHO)

It is the specialized agency of UNO. It was started in 1948 in order to help to achieve maximum level of health for all people. More than 100 countries are the members of WHO. It helps to finance its broad health activities throughout the world.

WHO has helped a great deal in the promotion of nursing education and practice in a number of ways, here in India. It has provided guidance in setting up program of nursing education and has promoted training for auxiliary nursing personnel. The WHO promotes public health in many ways around the world. Presently it is known for its declaration of working toward:

"Health for all by 2000 AD"

This declaration has given a tremendous impetus to develop primary health care and recognizing the very essential part of nursing in the health care system (Table 1).

Table 1: WHO has established subsidiary offices in various countries

Country	Office
Africa	Brazil
America	Washington
Eastern countries	Alexandria
Europe	Copenhagen, Denmark
South East Asia	New Delhi
Western Region Pacific	Manila, Philippines

World health day is celebrated in all member countries on 7th April each year and a theme is announced every year. Lectures and demonstrations are held to emphasize the bad effects of alcohol. Tobacco and other addiction forming elements. WHO adapted Alma-Ata Declaration, 'Health for all by 2000 AD' (Fig. 3).

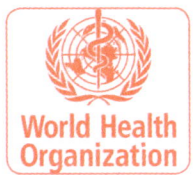

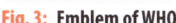

Fig. 3: Emblem of WHO

United Nations International Children's Emergency Fund (UNICEF)

This was established in 1946 previously known as UNICEF now called as UN Children Fund but keeps the title UNICEF. It works close collaboration with WHO. Headquarter of UNICEF is in New York and the regional office is in Delhi.

This institution is financed by governments of various countries, private institutions and individuals.

The main aim of UNICEF is to improve and promote the health of mother and children and facilitate programs to promote health of children.

The aim is fulfilled by participating in universe immunization program, providing primary care, taking care of child nutrition, family and child welfare and education and training.

UNICEF also provides ambulances, vehicles to the health department and dispensaries to facilitate health services in periphery. It also provides A-V aids and books to improve quality of nursing education.

UNICEF is an agency of the UNO (Fig. 4). It was founded in 1946 for the purpose of helping mothers and children in countries affected by World War II.

Today it offers services in all underdeveloped countries. It is financed by voluntary contributions from individuals and government.

The UNICEF has a great contribution in India. It provides teaching equipment for nursing education, Textbooks and visual aids for school of nursing and training for personnel for MCH services.

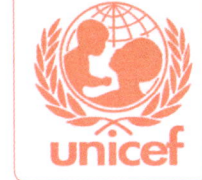

Fig. 4: Emblem of UNICEF

Functions of UNICEF

❑   It works for mother and child welfare and help the mother and child in emergency situations. This is achieved by the establishment of antenatal clinics, postnatal clinics and child welfare centers, under five or preschool clinics. It gives assistance to solve the problems of children all over the world.

❑   It provides ambulances, vehicle to health departments and dispensaries.

❑   It provides educational facilities for nurses and midwives. The nurses, training schools have been provided with equipment, audiovisual aids and textbooks.

GOBI Strategy

Currently UNICEF engaged in affecting the child's health revolution through GOBI campaign.

G – Growth monitoring

O – Oral dehydration therapy

B – Breastfeeding

I   – Universal immunization

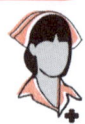

Red Cross Society

The Indian Red Cross Society is related to other Red Cross organizations around the world through international organization (Fig. 5). The important functions of this agency are:

- To protect human life at the time of disasters such as earthquakes, floods, cyclones and wars
- At the time of peace to protect the health of the population.
- To promote health by providing equipment and facilities to prevent diseases.

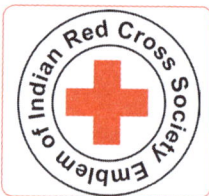

Fig. 5: Emblem of Indian Red Cross Society

Indian Red Cross Society has carried out the function of saving life at various times of national calamities as they arose in our country. This agency has provided medicines, equipment, medical experts, nurses and nursing assistants and sometimes the financial aid wherever necessary. It was presided by our then President of India Dr S Radhakrishnan. Executive body of this society has 21 members and a chairperson. Out of 21 members five members are nominated by the President of India.

Besides providing help at the time of national calamities, Indian Red Cross Society is still in process of providing assistance by the following ways:

- It supplies equipment to various hospitals, maternity centers, child welfare centers, schools and orphanages and helps other social welfare agencies in their work.
- In case of promoting maternal and child health, Red Cross Society contributes to a great extent. It provides modern equipment and medical facilities even in small villages particularly to those institutions which are devoted to particularly to those institutions which are devoted to maternal and child health work. The society prepares personal to carry out the function of giving medical and nursing aids and health education. It also provides training to public health nurses, trained dais, medical social workers and nursing personnel to look after crèches with help of government and social agencies available to the society. In 1959 it created a post of nursing staff officer and started home nursing training of health promoters who can give health education in local languages to the community.
- The Red Cross Society with the aim of providing health education particularly to those belonging to poor and backward strata of the society, brings out easily readable poster, pamphlet and booklets. It arranges film shows on personal hygiene, health for environment, causes and preventions of communicable and other diseases. It also brings out two monthly publications on the health matters which particularly emphasize health education of the community.
- Red Cross Society took the decision of training nurses in order to make nursing service available to the society. In 1959 it created a post of nursing staff officer and started home nursing training of health promoters who can give health education in local languages to the community.
- Indian Red Cross Society has created its own branch as junior Red Cross Society in the year 1926 which is actively working through young boys and girls in all over the country. The branch fulfills the objectives of promotion of health, and international fellowship.
- St John's Ambulance services also works along with Indian Red Cross Society in the country to take care of its various activities such as providing training in first aid to save life at the time of emergencies and to arrange for medical help as early as possible. It also trains personnel to undertake immunization program at the time of epidemics.

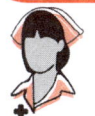

☐ Indian Red Cross Society has undertaken some other important activities in the field of health such as family welfare, by the way of family planning, supplying artificial limbs and equipment to physically handicapped, school supplementary nutrition program for the needy and establishment of blood bank to give blood for deserving and needy patients.

St John's Ambulance Association and St John Ambulance Brigade

This is the religious institution. The order of the hospitals of St John in England established St John Ambulance in 1877 with the specific aim of training persons to give first aid at the time of accidents and emergencies and to assist people to fight against sudden outbreak of diseases.

Functions of St John Ambulance Association and St John Ambulance Brigade

☐ To give care to the sick based on basic simple principles health care in the sick room in houses and educate public by visiting houses and spreading health advice.

☐ To train nurses and volunteers in first aid and care of the sick by establishing such institutions at different places in the country and send the health squads of volunteers and nurse wherever necessary at the places of disasters.

☐ To provide equipment required for the care of sick of giving first aid to the needy. It also provides ambulances to the factories, industrial belts, mines and at the time of mishaps and disaster.

☐ It provide health service to sick and wounded at time of peace in the country.

☐ The most important function is to train doctors, nurses and health workers and volunteers by conducting scientific and perfect training program particularly in first aid.

In India this organization is carrying out its functions independently and on voluntary basis from the year 1947 continuously.

It has also developed large membership in the country in its brigade and has organized ambulance services nursing and medical services and home guards services in country. The total membership is about 50,000, who have received training in first aid and primary care of the sick.

The international confederation of midwives (ICM) supports, represents and works to strengthen professional associations of midwives throughout the world. There are currently, 108 national midwives associations representing 95 countries across every continent. ICM is organized into four regions: Africa, The Americas, Asia Pacific and Europe. Together these associations represent more than 300,000 midwives globally.

ICM is an accredited non-governmental organization and represents midwives and midwifery worldwide to achieve common goals in care of mother and children. ICM works to strengthen midwives associations. It helps to enhance the reproductive health of women and new born.

Medical Association of India

Indian Medical Association is the only representative voluntary organization of doctors of modern scientific system of medicine in India, which looks after the interest of doctors as well as the well-being of the community at large. It was founded in 1928. Its head office is at Delhi.

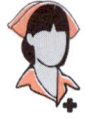

Colombo Plan

At Colombo in January, 1950 a meeting of the common wealth foreign ministers draw up a program for co-operative economic development in south and south east Asia. Membership comprises 20 developing countries within the region and six non-regional members. The main support of Colombo plan assistance goes for industrial and agricultural development but some support has also been given to health promotion mostly through fellowships. This plan provides for visits to countries by experts who can offer advice on local problems and train the local people. This plan is improving living standards of the people by reviewing developmental plans and co-ordinating development help.

World Bank

It is the specialized agency of the United Nations. It was establish with the purpose of helping less developed countries to arise their living standard. It provides financial and technical support for the projects of economic development.

The main objective of the World Bank is to help to raise the standards of living in comparatively poor and underdeveloped countries.

The main functions of World Bank are:

- ❑ Collaborates with WHO in supporting public health program on water supply
- ❑ Good production and pollution control
- ❑ AIDS control
- ❑ Generally, concerned with projects involving energy, transport, railway industries, education agriculture, family planning, health and environment etc.

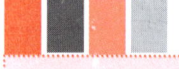 ASSESS YOURSELF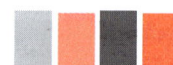

1. What do you mean by professional organization?
2. Write down the role of professional organizations in human welfare?

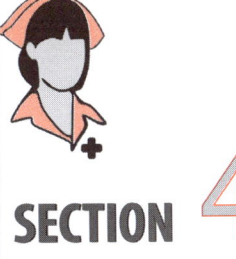

SECTION 4

NURSING ADMINISTRATION AND WARD MANAGEMENT

Introduction

17

Learning Objectives

- To discuss about the management.
- To describe the administration.
- To describe the administration and management of hospital and educational institutes.

Key Terms

- Prevoyance: Forecast and plan.
- Command: To lead.
- Managers: One who manages the work.

MANAGEMENT

- Management may be defined as the art of securing maximum results with a maximum of effort so as to secure maximum prosperity and happiness for both employer and employee and give the public the possible service. —**John Mee**
- Management is distinct process consisting of planning, organizing actuating, activating and controlling performed to determine and accomplish and objectives by the use of people and resources. —**George**

MANAGEMENT AND ADMINISTRATION

These two words are slightly similar and can employ interchangeable.

- Management refers to private sector whereas administration refers to public sector
- Management or administration is the process for exceeding the goal expected.
  —**Derek French and Heather Saward**

DIFFERENCE BETWEEN ADMINISTRATION AND MANAGEMENT

- Administration is concerned with policy making while management with policy implementation.

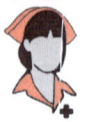

❏ Administration functions are legislative and largely determinative, whereas, that of management are executive and governing.

❏ Administration is concerned with planning and organizing whereas management's main concern is motivation and controlling.

❏ Board of directors of any organization or hospital is mainly concerned with administration, whereas personnel below that level are incharge of management.

WHO ARE MANAGERS?

Someone who coordinates and over as the work of other people so that organizational goals are accomplished.

Types of Managers (Fig. 1)

❏ **First-line managers:** Individual who manage the work of nonmanagerial employees.

❏ **Middle managers:** Individuals who manage the work of first-line managers.

❏ **Top managers:** Individuals who are responsible for making organization—wide decision and establishing plans and goals that affect the entire organization.

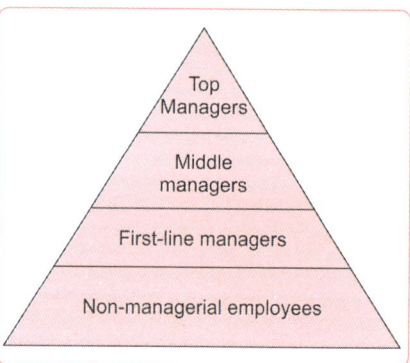

Fig. 1: Types of managers

Functions

❏ **Planning:** Defining goals, establishing strategies to achieve goals, developing plans to integrate and coordinate activities.

❏ **Organizing:** Arranging and structuring work to accomplish organizational goals.

❏ **Loading:** Working with and through people to accomplish goals.

❏ **Controlling:** Monitoring, comparing and correcting work.

Role

❏ **Interpersonal roles:** Figurehead, leader, liaison.

❏ **Informational roles:** Monitor, dissemination, spokesperson.

❏ **Decisional roles:** Entrepreneur, disturbance handle, resource allocator, negotiator.

Skills

❏ **Technical skills:** Knowledge and proficiency in a specific field.

❏ **Human skills:** The ability to work well with other people.

❏ **Conceptual skills:** The ability to think and conceptualize about abstract and complex situations concerning the organization.

Skills Needed at Different Management Levels (Fig. 2)

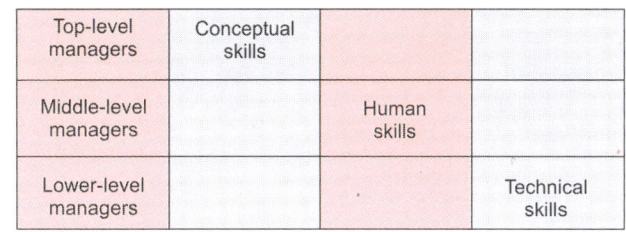

Top-level managers	Conceptual skills		
Middle-level managers		Human skills	
Lower-level managers			Technical skills

Fig. 2:   Different management levels

Importance of Management

The value of studying management:

❏ The universality of management
❏ Good management is needed in all organization
❏ The reality of work
❏ Employees either manage or are managed
❏ Rewards and challenges of being a manager
❏ Management offers challenging, exciting and creative opportunities for meaningful and fulfilling work
❏ Successful managers receive significant monetary rewards for their efforts.

ADMINISTRATION

Administration is a service, which engages in surveying planning, directing, executing maintaining and carrying to completion of a project   —**Large or small**

Administration derived from the Latin word 'ad' + 'ministrare', i.e. to care for or to look after people to manage affairs. Administration in the activities of groups co-operating to accomplish common goals.   —**Herbert A Simon**

Administration may be defined as the management of affairs with the use of well thought out principles and practices and rationalize techniques to achieve certain objectives.   —**Goel**

DEFINITIONS

Administration is the organization and direction of human and material resources to achieve desired ends.   — **Pfiffner and Presthus**

Administration has to do with getting things done; with the accomplishment of defined objectives.
                                                      —**Luther Gullick**

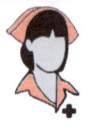

NATURE OF ADMINISTRATION (FIG. 3)

- ❑ Universal
- ❑ Holistic
- ❑ Intangible
- ❑ Continuous
- ❑ Goal oriented
- ❑ Social and human
- ❑ Dynamic
- ❑ Creative or innovative

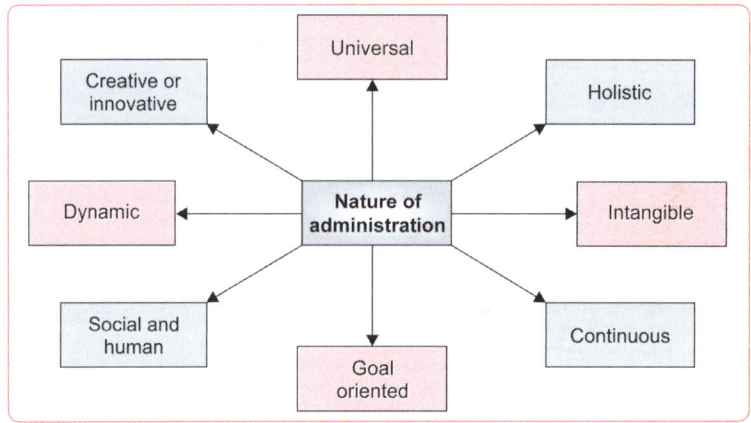

Fig. 3: Nature of administration

PHILOSOPHIES OF ADMINISTRATION

Philosophies of administration are based on the following key points:

- ❑ Cost effective
- ❑ Execution and control of work plans
- ❑ Delegation and responsibility
- ❑ Human relation and good morale
- ❑ Effective communication
- ❑ Flexibility in certain situation.

PRINCIPLES OF ADMINISTRATION AND MANAGEMENT

Meaning of management and administration principles: Management principles are statements of fundamental truth which act as guidelines for taking managerial action. Management principles are derived and developed in the following two steps:

1. Deep observation.
2. Repeated experiments.

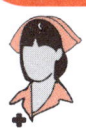

FAYOL'S 14 PRINCIPLES OF MANAGEMENT

1. **Division of work:** Specialization allows the individual to build up experience, and to continuously improve his skills. Thereby he can be more productive in small task, competent specialization, efficiency and effectiveness.
2. **Principle of authority and responsibility:** Authority means power to take decisions, responsibility and obligation to complete the job assigned.
3. **Principle of discipline:** General rules and regulations for systematic works in an organization.
4. **Principle of unity of command:** Employee should receive orders from one boss only.
5. **Unity of direction:** All the efforts of members and employees of the organization must be directed to one direction that is the achievement of common goal.
6. **Subordination of individual interest to general interest:** Subordination of individual interest to general interest of the organization must supersede the interest of the individuals.
7. **Principle of remuneration of persons:** Employees must be paid fairly or adequately to give them maximum satisfaction.
8. **Principle of centralization and decentralization:** Centralization refers to concentration of power in few hands. Decentralization is the division of power in many hands.
9. **Principle of scalar chain:** This means that line of authority should be from the highest rank to lowest rank.
10. **Principle of order:** Principle of order refers to orderly arrangement of man and material, a fixed place for everything and everyone in the organization.
11. **Principle of equity:** Fair and just treatment to employees.
12. **Stability of tenure of personnel:** Stability of tenure of personnel means there should not be frequent termination or transfer.
13. **Principle of initiative:** According to this principle the employees must be given opportunity to take some initiative in making and executing the plans.
14. **Principles of administration (Fig. 4):** According to Finer:

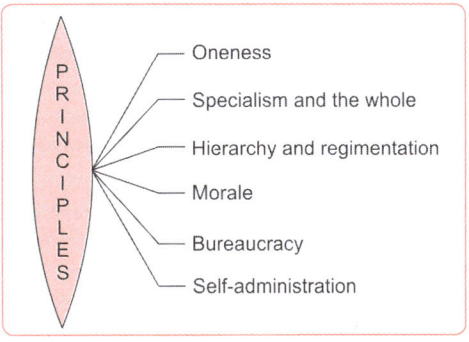

Fig. 4:   Administration principles

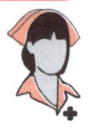

ELEMENTS OF ADMINISTRATION AND MANAGEMENT

According to Fayol's definition of management roles and actions distinguishes between five elements (Fig. 5). They are:

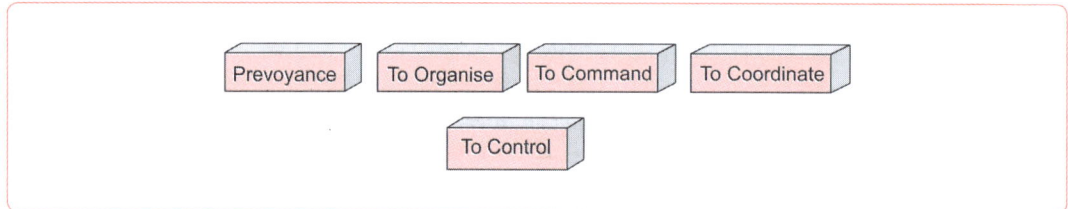

Fig. 5: Five elements of management

- ❏ **Prevoyance: (Forecast and Plan):** This element relates to the first step that is to examine the future and drawing up a plan of action and the elements of strategy.
- ❏ **To organize:** It is second element which tells about the buildup the structure means both, material and human of undertaking.
- ❏ **To command:** Maintain the activity among the personnel without command, management or administration is zero.
- ❏ **To coordinate:** Seeing that everything occurs in conformity with established rule and expressed command.

    Luther Gullick, an eminent management scientist classified management functions in an acronym POSDCORB
- ❏ **P** – Planning
- ❏ **O** – Organizing
- ❏ **S** – Staffing
- ❏ **D** – Directing
- ❏ **Co** – Coordinating
- ❏ **R** – Reporting
- ❏ **B** – Budgeting

SCOPE AND SIGNIFICANCE OF ADMINISTRATION AND MANAGEMENT

- ❏ **Political:** Function of administration includes the executive legislative relationship, so scope of the administration and management is vast in political area.
- ❏ **Defensive:** It covers the hospital protective function.
- ❏ **Economic:** Concerns with the vast area of the health care activities.
- ❏ **Educational:** It involves educational administration in the broadest senses.
- ❏ **Financial:** It includes the whole of financial, budget inventory control managements.
- ❏ **Social:** It includes the activities of the departments concerned with food, social factors.
- ❏ **Local:** It is concerned with the activities of the local bodies.

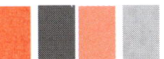 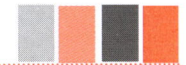 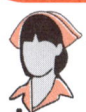

ASSESS YOURSELF

1. Define management. Describe the levels of management.

2. Define administration and throw light on nature of administration.

3. Discuss Fayol's 14 principles of management.

4. Write down in short elements of administration and management?

18 Management Process

Learning Objectives

📘 To discuss all aspects of management and administrations.
📘 To describe management process with its components.

Key Terms

- **Planning:** To organize something in a good manner in advance.
- **Organization:** Group of people having same goal.
- **Staffing:** To recruit and retain for work.
- **Control:** In limits.
- **Budgets:** Finance intake, output.

PLANNING

Planning is one of the major fundamental elements of administration. At planning stage, decisions are made about what needs to be done, how and when it has to be done by whom and with what resources. Planning is an intellectual process of making decisions and it aims to achieve a coordinated and consistent set of operations aimed at desired objectives. Any way for every work, management, administration, planning is must.

Definitions

Planning is a process of determining the objectives of administrative efforts and devising the means calculated to achieve them.
—Millet

Planning is a process of setting formal guidelines and constraints for the behavior of the person.
—Assoff and Brundinburg

Planning is a continuous process of making entrepreneurial decisions systematically and with the best possible knowledge for their future, organizing systematically the efforts needed to carry out these decision and measuring the result of the decision against expectations though systematic feedback.
—Drucher

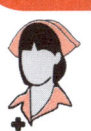

Importance

Planning is considered important because:

- It attempts to offset uncertainty by foreseeing the future and bringing about preparedness for the happening in the future.
- It focuses attention on the objectives or goals of the organization and their achievement.
- It leads to economy in operation through the selection of the best possible course of action.
- It helps in controlling the activities by providing measures against which performance can be evaluated.
- It helps in coordinating the operations of an organization.

Principles

- Planning must focus on purposes. It should always be based on clearly defined objectives.
- Planning is a continuous and iterative process which includes series of steps, so continuity and flexibility should be maintained in planning cycle.
- Planning should be simple and there should be provision for proper analysis and clarification of actions.
- In planning there should be good harmony with organization and environment, political as well as economical etc.
- Planning is hierarchical in nature and must have an organizational identification.
- Planning should be pervasive activity covering the entire organization with all its departments, sectors and different levels of administration, and it should be balanced.
- Planning must be precise in its objective scope and nature. It should be realistic in its scope and pinpoint the expected result.
- In planning the provision should be made to use all available resources.
- Planning should always be documented so that all the concerned are fully committed to the implementation of the program.

Characteristics (Fig.1)

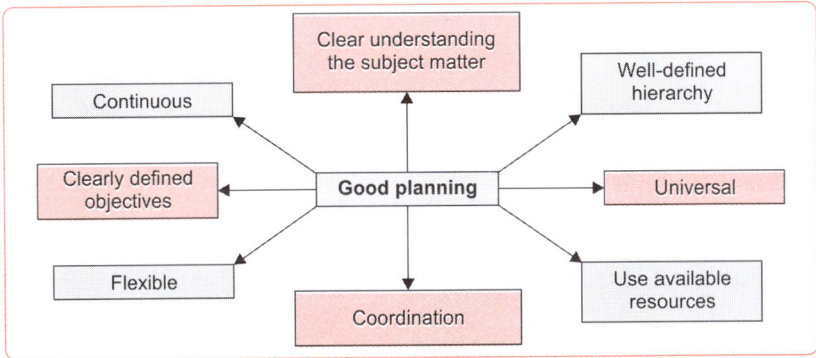

Fig: 1   Good planning

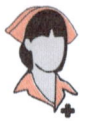

RC Davis has described six features of good planning:

1. Plan should have specific objectives and there objectives should be known to every member who so ever are engaged in planning.
2. Planning should be flexible.
3. Planning should have well-explained rationale behind it.
4. Planning should be universal, simple and economical.
5. It should be stabilizing.
6. Planning should be continues and should be made according to the need of future.

Components/Elements (Fig. 2)

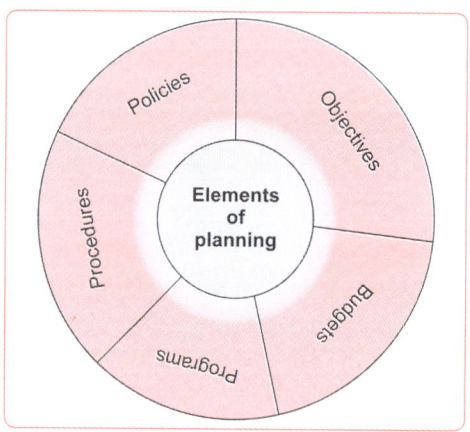

Fig. 2: Elements of planning

- **Objectives:** Objectives are basic plans which determine goals or end results of the projected action of an enterprise by setting goals. Objectives provide the foundation upon which structure of plan can be built.
- **Policies:** Policies are written statements or oral understanding. In some, they are general terms for governing actions in repetitive situations. Realization of objectives is made easy with the help of policies, as policies provide standing solution to problem.
- **Procedures:** Procedures indicate the specific manner in which a certain activity is to be performed. They are more definite and specific guides to action, but only for fulfillment of objectives.
- **Program:** Programs weld together different plans for implementing them into completely and orderly course of action. Programs are necessary for both repetitive (routine planning) and nonrepetitive (creative planning) course of action.
- **Budgets:** Budgets are plans continuing statements of expected results in numerical terms, i.e. rupees, man hours, product units and so forth.

Steps (Flow chart 1)

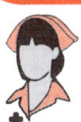

Flow chart 1: Steps of planning

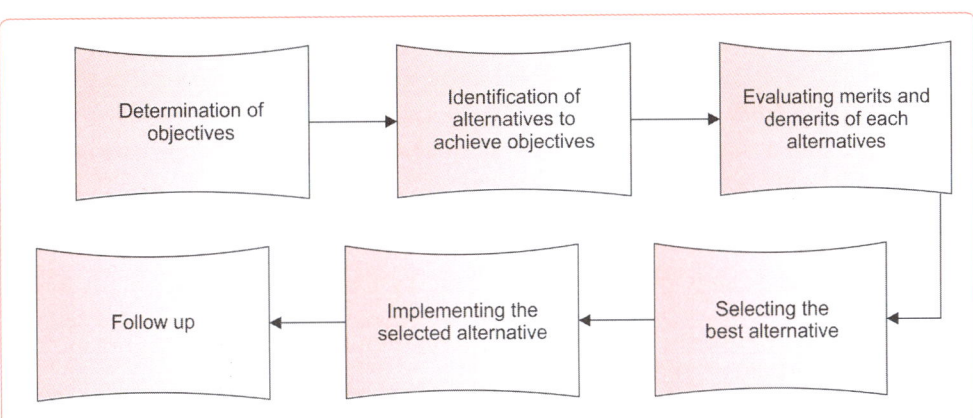

- **Determination of objectives:** Major objectives are broken into departmental, sectional and individual objectives. These must be spelled out in realistic and specific terms.
- **Establishment of planning premises:** Planning premises supply pertinent facts and information relating to the future and as such they are vital to the success of planning.
- **Selection of operative plan from alternatives:** In other words the techniques of decision making are applied to choose the proposed course of action from several alternatives. If alternatives are not developed, planning becomes a straight jacket pattern of activity and poses much of its beneficial result.
- **Implementation of the selected alternatives:** The selected alternative should be implemented. It should be flexible enough to adjust to changed conditions and to unusual and unexpected situation.
- **Follow-up and evaluation:** Since all pertinent facts are not available in most planning activities and since some guess work in inevitable, there should be a prior provision for following up the proposed program when it is put into action. For this, one should have regular feedback both the way by written records and by direct observation. Evaluation is measuring what has been done against what had been planned to do.

Types

Planning must be done at several levels and each has its own particular problems and configuration of the planners and methods. The planning can be classified as follows:

Directional Planning

It is often called policy planning and is concerned with broad general direction of the program, i.e. setting the framework of intent and philosophy within which the program will proceed, and with selecting the program to the broad planning of the community in which the program will function.

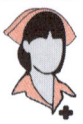

Administrative Planning

It is concerned with the overall implementation of the policies developed and with mobilization and coordination of the personnel and material available in the administrative unit for the effectuation of the service.

Operational Planning

It is concerned with actual delivery of the service to the community. Planning may be classified as long range and short range and also strategic and operation planning.

Strategic Planning

❑ Usually it is long range planning and is done by the top level managers. It includes the following activities.
   ▪ SWOT (analysis of strengths, weakness, opportunities and threats) of organization both internal and external environment
   ▪ Developing philosophy and formulation of policies and objectives on basis of analysis of the organization
   ▪ Allocation of resources on the basis of priority
   ▪ Evaluation of activities to increase efficiency
   ▪ Providing proper direction to avoid duplication of service.

Operational Planning

Usually this is operational and short range planning and is undertaken by middle or supervisory level personnel.
❑ Planning for a few months to a financial year.
❑ Planning for details budgeting, provision for short range goods and it should be achieved within a given period
❑ Extensional aspect of long range plan.

Planning Process in Health Service or Planning Cycle (Fig. 3)

Planning process or planning cycle can be explained in eight steps as follows:
1. Assessing the planning environment which means none of the environment and socioeconomic cultural peculiarities.
2. Data collection using rapid, rural appraisal technique where necessary and data analysis for bringing out the problems and potentials of the area.
3. Strategy formulation and setting realistic targets for the plan.
4. Participatory plan formulation.
5. Plan authentication and linking the plan with the plan at the near higher level.
6. Task adoption and plan implementation.
7. Mid-term appraisal and make corrections.
8. Evaluation and replanning.

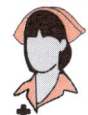

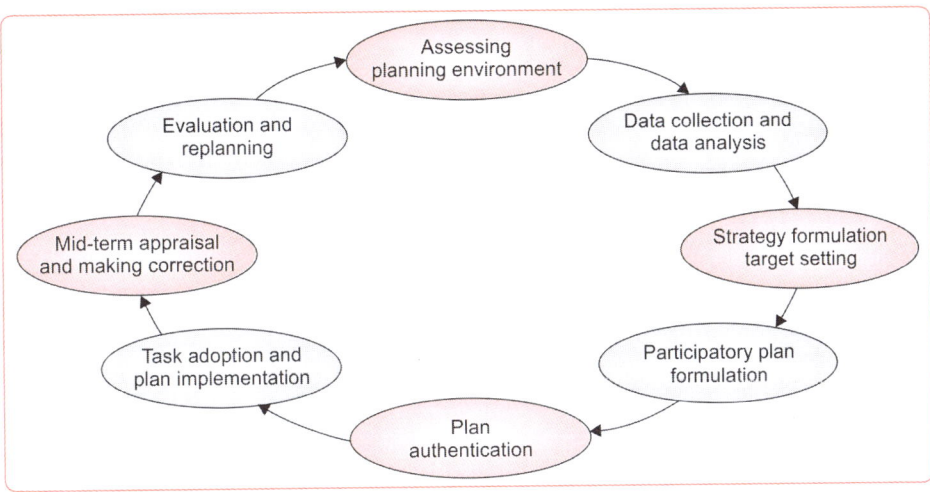

Fig. 3:   Planning cycle and planning process

ORGANIZATION

An organization is an establishment of the formal structure of authority through which the work is sub-divided, arranged, defined and coordinated for defined objectives. An organization is made to run an institution. Nothing can be accomplished in a proper way without organization.

Definitions

❑ Organization is a form of human association for the attainment of common purpose.

—*JB Moorey*

❑ Organization can be defined as a process of identifying and grouping the work to be performed. Defining and delegating responsibility and authority, and establishing relationship for the purpose of enabling people to work together most effectively in accomplishing the objectives.

❑ Organizational structure is a pattern of interrelated posts connected by the authority.

—*Milward*

❑ Organization is the formal structure of authority through which subdivisions are arranged, defined and coordinated for defined objectives.

Types

There are many types of the organizations. In fact it is a process of dividing and combining the activities. It may be of any type but has to organize the four 'Ps' these are....

❑ P – Purpose, function
❑ P – Process
❑ P – Person, clientele
❑ P – Place, setting

The main types of the organization are as follows:

❑ Formal organization
❑ Nonformal organization

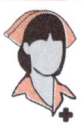

- ❑ Informal organization
- ❑ Line organization
- ❑ Staff organization
- ❑ Line and staff organization
- ❑ Committee organization
- ❑ Social organization

Principles

The following are the principles of organization:

- ❑ **Authority and responsibility:** Authority is the right or power to give orders to the subordinates whereas responsibility in the duty which the subordinate is expected to perform by virtue of its position in the organization. There should be a perfect balance between authority and responsibility.
- ❑ **Hierarchy:** Hierarchy means the rule or control of the higher to lower. Hierarchy consists in the universal application of the superior–subordinate relationship through a number of levels of responsibility from the top to the bottom of structure.
- ❑ **Division of labor:** This is the principle of specialization which applies to all kinds of work. The more people specialize, the more efficiently they can perform their work. This principle is equally applicable to managerial work as to technical work.
- ❑ **Discipline:** Discipline means getting obedience to rules and regulations of the organization. Discipline is necessary for the smooth running of the organization. Good discipline is the result of effective leadership. A clear understanding between management and works regarding the organization's rule and the judicious use of penalties for violation of rules.
- ❑ **Unity of command:** No one can make happy to two masters. This proverb tells us about the importance of unity of command. This principle emphasizes that one subordinates should receive orders from one superior only as dual command is permanent source of conflict. Therefore, in every organization each subordinate should have one superior whose command he has to obey.
- ❑ **Unity of direction:** It is the condition essential to the unity of action. Coordination of strength and focusing of efforts. Unity of direction is provided by sound organization of the body corporate, unity of command cannot exist without unity of direction. This principle to mean one head and one plan for group of activities having the same objectives.
- ❑ **Coordination:** Coordination in every organization between various departments and within the departments' activities are indispensable to achieve the desired objectives. Lack of coordination causes tremendous waste of time, effort and money.
- ❑ **Centralization versus decentralization:** Centralization stands for concentration of authority at or near top. An organization is said to be centralized if most of the power of decision is vested in the top level so that the lower ones have to refer most problems to the head of the organization and his immediate subordinates for decision.

  Decentralization means that the central authority gives certain powers to the local authorities. A decentralized organization is one in which the lower levels are allowed the discretion to decide most of the matters which come up reserving comparatively a few bigger and more important problem only for those higher up.

  Neither centralization nor decentralization can be accepted in an absolute principle of good organization under these circumstances.

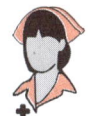

❑ **Integration and disintegration:** Administrative bench should be fully integrated. Integration means unification in administrative language. According to integration principle, several administrative units combine together to make a single whole organization. While under disintegration, every service is treated as an independent unit in itself and bear no direct relation with each other, under integrated administration, whole administration is centered in one and he is the chief executive. But in the disintegrated administration constitution vests in individual departments right and authority to act freely.

Need/Importance

❑ Organization is required for utilization of the ability and productive capacity of the workers.
❑ The main aim of organization structure is to put the right man on the right job on the basis of one's specialized qualification, experience, talent and aptitude.
❑ Facilitates efficiency and effectiveness of the organization.
❑ Provides path way for communication.
❑ Helps in optimum use of human resources.
❑ Encourages creativity of the workers.
❑ Organization's structure facilitates growth of institution.
❑ Helps in proper use of resources.
❑ Facilitates in determining the responsibility and authority of each department and personnel working in it in a better way.
❑ Facilitates in defining the position and role to be played by each member in the organization.
❑ Provides channels of communication which will help in the coordination among members and determine the number of subordinates who should report directly to each manager/superiors.
❑ Decides at which level various types of decision are to be taken.

Importance of organization can be shown as given in Figure 4:

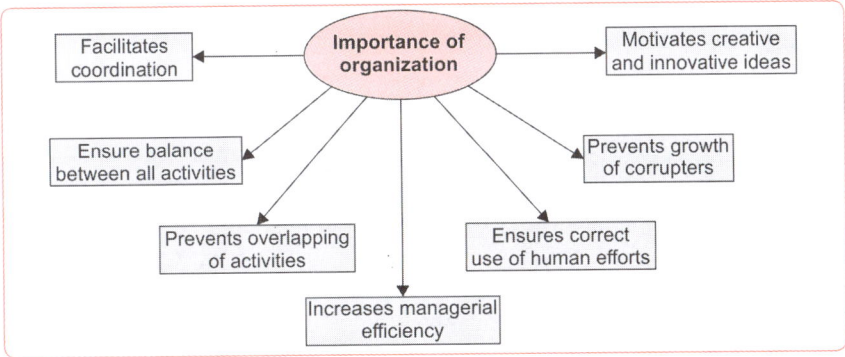

Fig. 4: Importance of organization

Organizational Structure

Organizational structure can be expressed in flow charts which show the levels of organization. Flow charts 2 to 7 are given in this chapter which is self-explanatory in nature:

❑ Basic organizational service plan for hospital nursing
❑ District health organizational chart
❑ Organizational chart of ward

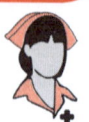

❑ Organizational chart for PHC
❑ Organizational chart for subcenter

Flow chart 2: **Basic organization plan for hospital nursing services**

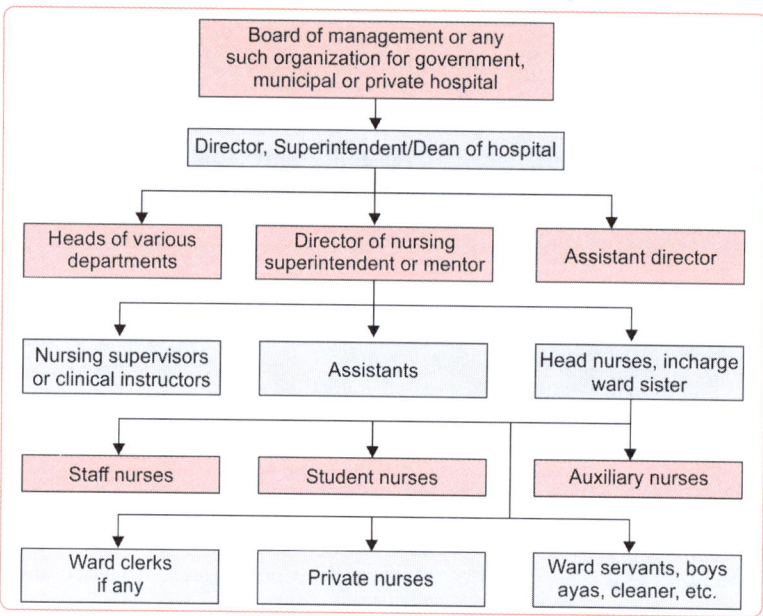

Flow chart 3: **District health organizational chart**

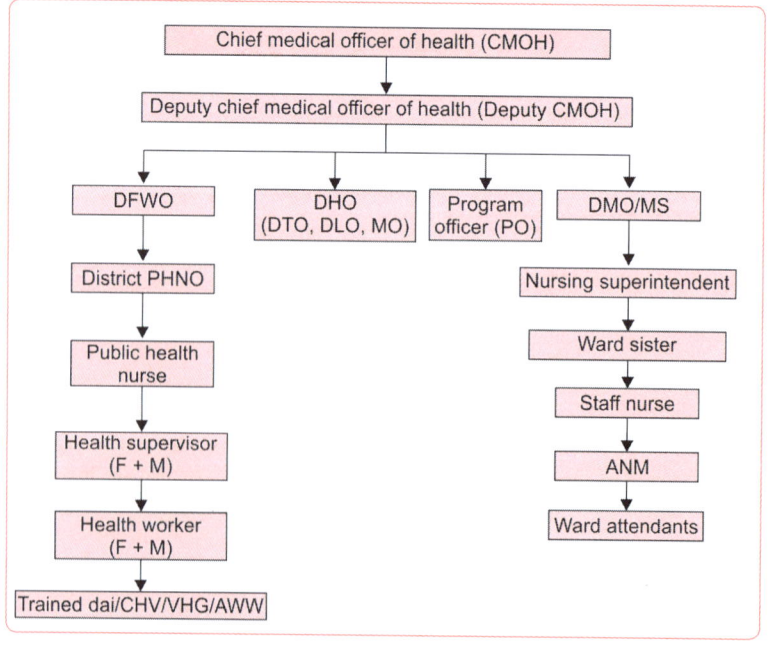

Abbreviations

PO	—	Program Officer
DFWO	—	District Family Welfare Officer
DHO	—	District Health Officer
DTO	—	District Tuberculosis Officer
DLO	—	District Leprosy Officer
MO	—	Malaria Officer
DMO	—	District Medical Officer
Dt PHN	—	District Public Health Nurse
PHN	—	Public Health Nurse
CHV	—	Community Health Volunteer
VHG	—	Village Health Guide
AWW	—	Anganwadi Worker
MS	—	Medical Superintendent
PHNO	—	Public Health Nursing Officer

PHN	—	Public health nurse
CHC	—	Community health center
PHC	—	Primary health center
LHV	—	Lady health visitor
HS	—	Hidradenitis suppurativa (House supervision)
ANS	—	Assistant nursing superintendent
ANM	—	Auxiliary nurse midwife

Levels and Population
- District level: 10–15 million
- Block level: 60–80 thousand
- Section level: 15–25 thousand
- Subcenter level: 3.5–8 thousand
- Village level: 1–3 thousand

Flow chart 4: **Organizational chart of hospital**

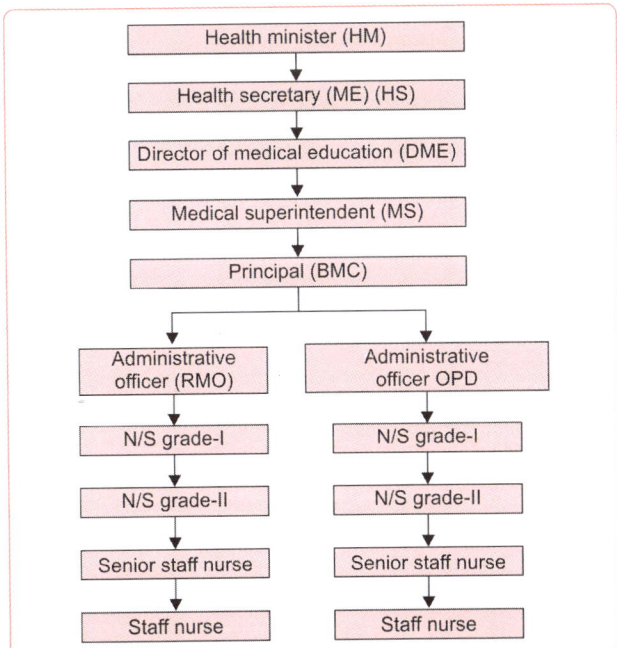

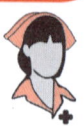

Flow chart 5: Organizational chart of a ward

ANS
Ward sister N/S grade-I
Ward sister N/S grade-I
Nursing sister grade-II
Supporting staff
Senior staff nurse
Staff nurse
ANM
Student nurse

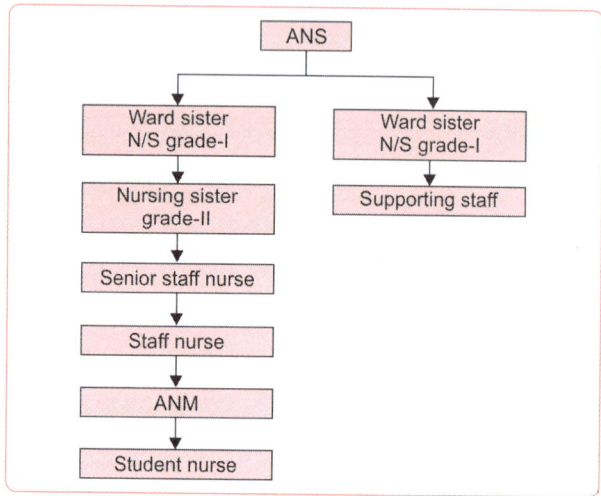

Flow chart 6: Organizational chart of PHC

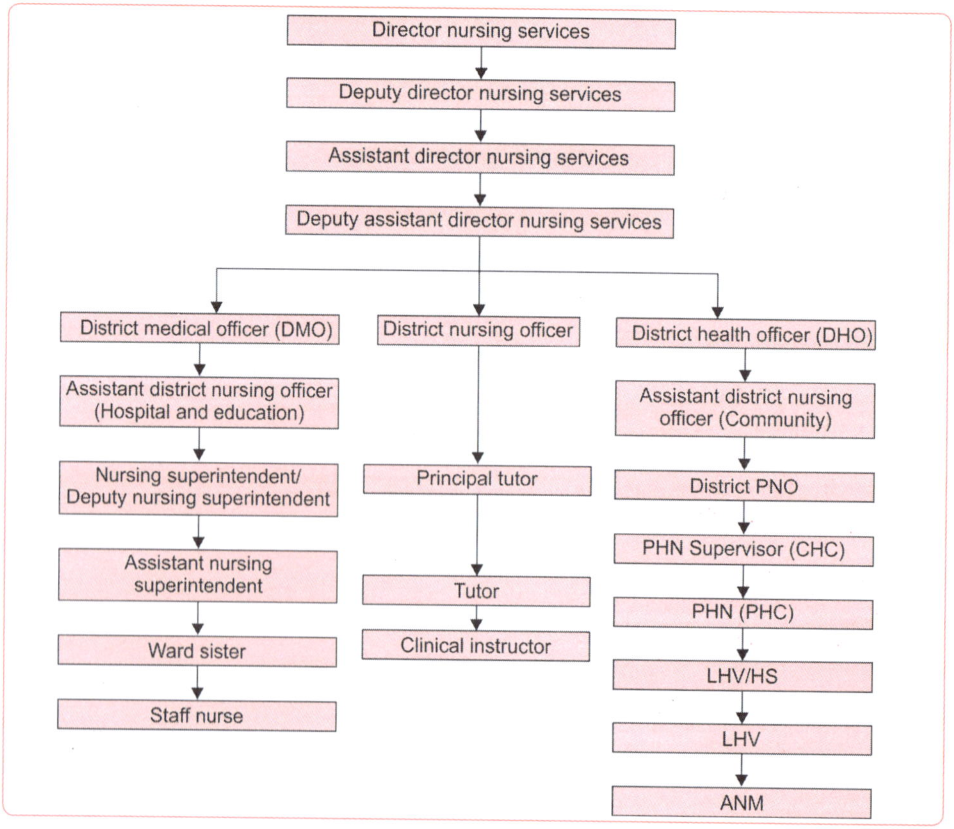

Director nursing services
Deputy director nursing services
Assistant director nursing services
Deputy assistant director nursing services
District medical officer (DMO)
District nursing officer
District health officer (DHO)
Assistant district nursing officer (Hospital and education)
Assistant district nursing officer (Community)
Nursing superintendent/ Deputy nursing superintendent
Principal tutor
District PNO
PHN Supervisor (CHC)
Assistant nursing superintendent
Tutor
PHN (PHC)
Ward sister
Clinical instructor
LHV/HS
Staff nurse
LHV
ANM

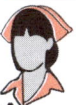

Flow chart 7: **Organizational chart of subcenter**

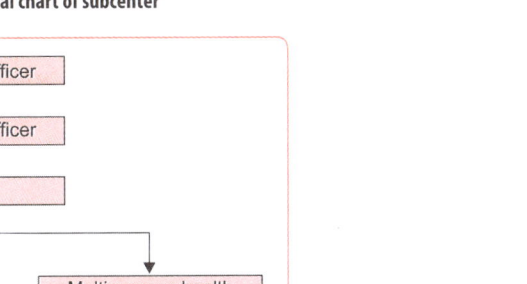

STAFFING

Introduction

Having known the functions to be performed by a particular type of individual or group of individuals, right persons are recruited. Staffing as a management function involves recruiting, selection, development through training, retaining, promotion and retirement of human resources in an organization.

Meaning

The term staffing pertains to number and composition of personnel assigned to work on a unit at a given time.

Purpose

The purpose of staffing patterns is appropriate coverage of the job to be done in the interest of the patients entrusting themselves to be institution and equitable utilization of nurses in their interest.

Factors Influencing Staffing Pattern

Staffing is concerned with manpower planning and development in order to ensure that requisite number of staff with appropriate skills is employed at the right time to meet the requirement of the work to be done. Staffing patterns are influenced by wide variety of mutually dependent factors within any situation. Some factors are as follows:

❑   Types of nursing services
❑   Number of patients
❑   Standard of care

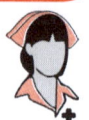

❑ Role defined by profession
❑ Qualification and job specification
❑ Supply of personnel
❑ Patient condition, ICU
❑ Fluctuation of work load
❑ Method of assignment
❑ Geography of nursing unit
❑ Supporting staff
❑ Type of hospital

Staffing Requirement/Scheduling

Staffing schedule for school/college and hospitals for nursing is fixed by the authorities (Table 1). As staffs for schools/college of nursing is as per norms of Indian Nursing Council.

❑ One nurse teacher to 10 students school of nursing/college of nursing.
❑ Staff for management position at directorate level
❑ Lower staff for maintenance

Table 1: Nursing staff for hospital (wards, special units and OPD)

Ward	Staff nurse	Ward sister	Departmental sister
Medical ward	1:3	1:25	1 for 3–4 wards
Surgical ward	1:3	1:25	
Orthopedic ward	1:3	1:25	
Pediatric ward	1:3	1:25	
Gynecological ward	1:3	1:25	
Maternity ward (including newborns)	1:3	1:25	
ICU	1:1	1 each	1 departmental sister
CCU	1:1	1 each	
Nephrology	1:1	1 each	
Neurology	1:1		
Special wards	1:1	3–4 units together	1 departmental sister
Operation theater	3:1 (1 table)	1 for each shift	
Casualty and emergency	2:3		
Assistant nursing superintendent	1:150 beds	1 each shift	
Ward sister/supervisor	1:25 beds	1 for each shift	
Staff nurse for wards	1:3 + 30% leave reserve		
Nurse in OPD and emergency			

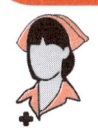

Staffing Formulae

$$\text{Number of hours required or recommended for staff development per year per person} \times \text{Number of staff} = \text{Number of hours per year for staff development needing relief coverage}$$

$$\text{Number of staff development hours needing coverage} \div \text{Hours worked/day} \div \text{Total days worked/person} = \text{Full time personnel required for staff development coverage}$$

RECRUITMENT

Recruitment has become the most challenging human resource management (HR) function and it is one of the activities that impact more critically on the performance of an organization. Recruiting strategy must follow certain consideration, like aggressive growth plans, retention, recruit costs, time factor, intellectual property, impact on quality and safety.

Well-planned and well-managed recruiting efforts will result in high quality applicants. Acquiring and retaining the employees is high quality talent and critical to an organization success. and organize need to analyze the benefits and disadvantages of recruiting its personnel through internal or external sources and whether formal or informal system will be used.

Poor recruitment decision continues to affect organizational performance, limit goal achievement and also can produce long-term negative effects among them.

Definitions

"The set of activities and process used to legally obtain a sufficient number of qualified people at right place and right time, such that people and the organization can select each other in their own best short- and long-term interest."

"The process of searching for and obtaining application for jobs, from among the right people can be selected."

"The recruitment process provides the organization with a pool of potentially qualified job candidates from which judicious selection can be made to fill the vacancies."

"Recruitment refers to the process of attracting, screening, and selecting a qualified person for job."

Purposes

- ❑ Provide pool of potentially qualified applicants for job
- ❑ Select the suitable candidate for job
- ❑ Determine the present and future requirements of the organization in conjunction with its personnel planning and job analysis activities
- ❑ Enhance success rate of the selection process
- ❑ Limit under qualified or over qualified job applicants

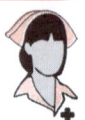

- Retains the employee for long time
- Meet the organizations legal and social obligations regarding the composition of its workforce
- Increase organizational and individual effectiveness in short-term and long-term
- Evaluate the effectiveness of various recruiting techniques and sources for all types of job applicants
- Recruitment is the process which links the employers with the employees.

Factors Affecting Recruitment

Recruitment differs according to:

- Size of the organization
- Employment condition in the community
- Effect of the past recruitment efforts
- Working condition and salary or other benefits
- Rate of growth of organization
- Cultural, economical and legal aspects.

Recruitment Strategies

Each organization has a human resource management department. Its main function is recruitment. Recruitment means to employ the deserved person legally on the right job, because the performance of the organization directly depends upon the employees who are recruited. A good and well planned programmed strategy is needed to recruit the talent and to motivate the talent to apply for the organization. A good strategy should have the following elements:

- **Identifying the jobs:** In every organization a number of jobs are there which are to be filled according to the priority of the area. It is a never ending process. The human resource department has to identify and prioritize the job in the different areas and see whether it is a real need or not. They have to focus on the key jobs first.
- **Candidates:** Once the need of job is identified then one has to see which type of the candidate is required to fulfill the conditions of the job. What type of parameters the person should have? Some of the parameters may be as follows:
  - **Performance level required:** Different strategies are required for focusing on hiring high performers and average performers.
  - **Experience level required:** The strategy should be clear as to what is the experience level required by the organization. The candidate's experience can range from being a fresher to experienced senior professionals.
  - **Category of the candidate:** The strategy should clearly define the target candidate. He/she, can be from the same industry, different industry, unemployed, top performers of the industry, etc.
- **Sources of recruitment:** The strategy should define various sources (external and internal) of recruitment. Which are the sources to be used and focused for the recruitment purposes for various positions? Employee referral is one of the most effective sources of recruitment.

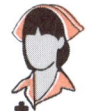

❑ **Trained recruiters:** The recruitment professionals conducting the interviews and the other recruitment activities should be well-trained and experienced to conduct the activities. They should also be aware of the major parameters and skills (e.g. behavioral, technical, etc.) to focus while interviewing and selecting a candidate.

❑ **How to evaluate the candidates:** The various parameters and the way to judge them, i.e. the entire recruitment process should be planned in advance. Like the rounds of technical interviews, HR interviews, written tests, psychometric tests, etc.

Recruitment Process

The process of finding and attracting capable applicants for employment, it will inform qualified individual about jobs and employment opportunities. Create positive image of organization, so the applicants can make comparison with their qualification, interest and generate enthusiasm, interest among the candidates.

Process includes:

❑ Identify vacancy
❑ Prepare job description and person specification
❑ Advertising the vacancy
❑ Managing the response
❑ Short-listing
❑ Arrange interviews
❑ Conducting interview and decision making.

The recruitment process is immediately followed by the selection process, i.e. the final interviews and the decision making, conveying the decision and the appointment formalities.

Recruitment Methods

Recruitment for the talented employees is must to run an organization smoothly. The agencies use multiple methods to recruit the needy employees as follows:

❑ **Advertising:** Advertisement in local, national, regional newspaper, journals, cable television's employment news, etc. Advertisement should be eye catching, clear, and should be designed in such a way to attract talent.

❑ **Employment agencies:** There are a number of agencies which provides employment to the deserving candidates. They in fact help the both, employees as well as the organization.

❑ **Career day programs:** There are number of joins which are organized to attract the employees. Sometimes campus recruitments are also done.

❑ **Through database:** Maintain a database or filling system for potential employees based on resumes.

- Qualification
- Experience
- Physical fitness
- Category of the candidate etc.

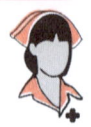

Sources of Recruitment

Now the stage comes that from where the talent can be searched so the sources are the only option. The sources may be internal or external. It may be referral services.

- ❑ **Training of the new talent:** Each organization has its own type and line of work. The strategy has to make for conducting interviews and other recruitment activities like written test, fitness test or practical test. They should be aware of other parameters like behavioral, technical skills, etc.
- ❑ **Evaluation of candidate:** One should have a parameter or a scale to evaluate the candidate for the recruitment. Which should be in black and white? A web site of the organization should be there to help the potential candidates.
- ❑ **Internal recruitments:** The personnel/employees already working in the organization can be recruited for the post. It may be a type of promotion or transfer from one post to other post. This books the motivation of the employees.
- ❑ **Employee referrals:** The already selected employees help to recruit the talent from their known, near ones. That may attract the talent from the other organizations. The friends of the employees working are not satisfied with the organization they work for, so existing employees can be a great source for hunting the talent for new vacancy.

Credentialing

The process of establishing the qualification of licensed professionals is called or known as credentialing. Many health care institutions and provider networks conduct their own credentialing. It is the value free name of a variable that is known to be a reliable indicator of quality that is known to be a reliable indicator of quality.

It may include granting and reviewing specific clinical privileges and medical, health staff membership.

Educational and Credential Requirement

Consideration should be given to educational requirement and credentials for each job category as long as relationship exist between these requirement and success on job. If requirement for a position are too rigid, they may remain unfilled for some time.

Sometimes people who are able to complete credential or educational requirement may deny the opportunity to complete the job. Therefore, many organizations have a list of preferred criteria for a position and a second list of minimal criteria.

SELECTION

After applicants have been recruited, have completed their applications, and have been interviewed, the next step in the employment staffing process is selection.

Definition

Selection is the process of choosing from applicants the best qualified individual for a particular job or position.

The process involves verifying the applicant's qualification, checking his/her work history, and deciding if a good match exist between the applicant's qualification and the organizations expectations (Flow chart 8).

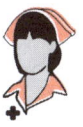

Flow chart 8: **Selection process**

```
              ┌──────────────────────────┐
              │   Adequate applicant pool │
              └────────────┬─────────────┘
                           ↓
              ┌──────────────────────────┐
              │  Pre-employment screening │
              └────────────┬─────────────┘
                           ↓
              ┌──────────────────────────┐
              │ Completion of application │
              └────────────┬─────────────┘
       ┌──────────┬────────┴───────┬───────────────┐
       ↓          ↓                ↓               ↓
┌───────────┐ ┌─────────────┐ ┌───────────┐ ┌────────────┐
│ Reference │ │Pre-employment│ │ Physical  │ │ Employment │
│  checks   │ │  testing    │ │examination│ │ interview  │
└───────────┘ └─────────────┘ └─────┬─────┘ └────────────┘
                                     ↓
                          ┌────────────────────┐
                          │  Employer decision  │
                          └──────────┬─────────┘
                                     ↓
                          ┌────────────────────┐
                          │   Notification of   │
                          │     applicants      │
                          └────────────────────┘
```

Reference Checks

All applicants should be examined to see if they are complete and to ascertain that the applicant is qualified for the position. At this point, references are requested and employments history is verified.

Clearly a strong application and excellent reference do not necessarily guarantee excellent job performance: however carefully reviewing application and checking references may help to prevent bad hiring decision.

Occasionally, reference calls will reveal unsolicited information about the applicant. Information obtained by any informant may not be used to reject an applicant unless a justifiable reason for disqualification exists.

Re-employment Testing

To test the ability of the applicant to perform a specific job re-employment testing is used although it alone is not a tool for selection. It is joined with other tools like physical examination, interview, etc.

Physical Examination

This is also a selection tool especially for the recruitment where the person has to perform the physical job, e.g. in army, police, etc. Each organization want that the employee who takes job should be physically fit so the physical examination for fitness for the selected job in must. If the person is not physically fit for the job that application can be rejected.

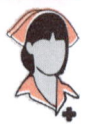

Employment Interview

Interview is the face to face or telephonically interaction between the two or more persons. It is the most common form of selection. It is beneficial for both employer and the candidate are as follows:

For the employer:

- Information given in the application can be confirmed.
- Communication skills can be judged.
- Reactions to the situations can be judged by employer.
- Other personal queries can be cleared.

For the candidate:

- Candidate can judge the environment where he/she has to work.
- Candidate can see whether he/she can merge in the working culture of the organization
- Candidate can put up his/her expectations.

Making the Selection

When determine the most appropriate person to hire, the manager must be sure that the same standards are used to evaluate all candidates. Final selection should be based on established criteria not on value or personal judgment.

For both internal and external applicants same interview procedure or criteria for selection should be used, some organization give special consideration and preferences to their own employee. Every organization should have some guidelines and criteria how promotion and transfers are to be handled.

Finalizing the Selection

Once a final selection has been made, manager should be responsible for closure of the re-employment process:

- The decision should be informed to the candidate as the final selection is made.
- Changes if any in position or other facts should be notified as soon as possible with the appropriate reasons.
- If any misunderstanding or conflict occurs then it should be cleared before joining the job.
- Applicants or candidates who are selected should be requested to confirm in writing their intention to accept the post.

PLACEMENT

Placement means to get the right man at right place and right job to fulfill the objectives of the organization. It is a way to assigning rank according to the expectation of the candidate and the requirement of the organization. The supervisor took the responsibility to find out that the person is properly fit.

If the candidate feels that the placement is not proper or according to the expectations, decision and remedy, the situation without delay should be done.

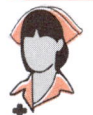

PROMOTION

The word promotion is derived from the Latin word 'promover' means "to move forward". It is a positive appraisal. It is the term which refers to a change for better prospects from one job to another job in deemed by employee. Generally unions favor promotions on the basis of seniority or the basis of merit. The opposition of the promotion is demotion.

Certain guidelines must be accompanying promotion selection to ensure that the process is fair and equitable. The following elements should be determined in advance:

❑ Whether the recruitment will be internal or external
❑ What the promotion and selection criteria will be
❑ The adequate pool of candidates
❑ Handling rejected candidates
❑ How employees released are to be handled?

JOB DESCRIPTION

The collected job data is quantify and processed through a computer. After weighing the job content and working conditions a formal job description and specification should be written.

Definition

Job description is a clear, concisely and clearly communicating written statement of duties and responsibilities and organizational relationships that constitute a given job or position.

Job description refers to requirements for a particular job position. The requirements include skill requirements, the level of experience needed, and level of education required, roles and responsibilities attached with the job position.

The job description usually covers the following information:

❑ **Job title and location:** It includes the title of job/description department, code number.
❑ **Job summary:** It is a brief write up about the job.
❑ **Job activities/duties:** The description of task done, facilities used, etc.
❑ **Working conditions:** The physical environment, any hazards, etc.
❑ **Work environment:** The size of work group, work culture, interpersonal interaction, etc.
❑ **Performance standards:** The standards required for the personal to evaluate for the performance.

Importance and Purpose

❑ Job description help the nurse applicant know about the duties and responsibilities with a particular job position and clarify work function.
❑ It facilitates the nurse employee to understand properly the requirements of job and gives a summary of important functions and expectations of particular job positions to a potential employ.
❑ It aids in job evaluation.
❑ It provides basis for manpower planning.
❑ It assists in recruitment, selection, placement, orientation career planning and evaluation of nurse employee.

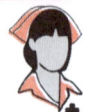

- It also helps in bench marking the performance standards.
- It helps for classifying the levels of nursing functions according to the skill levels.
- Helps to identify training needs of nurse.
- Serve as a channel of communication.
- Helps in job evaluation.
- It helps in maintaining nurse employees discipline.
- It helps in work scheduling.

A job description should be very clear, concise and should have the following information:

- Job title and location
- Job summary
- Job duties
- Educational qualifications
- Skills and specifications
- Working conditions

Job description should be given to every employee so that the employee should know what ever he/she has to do.

JOB SPECIFICATION

Job specification is a written statement of qualifications, traits, physical and mental characteristics that an individual must possess as a minimum requirement to perform the job duties and discharge responsibilities effectively and satisfactory. It specifies the types of person required on the job and further assists in the selection of appropriate personnel by outlining the particular working conditions to be encountered on the job. It describes the extent to which compensable factors as education, experience, efforts, physical demand, etc. exist in a particular job.

A statement of personal qualifications necessary to do the job usually contains such items as education, experience training, judgment, initiative, physical effort, skills, responsibilities communication skills, emotional characteristics, mental health, special attributes and abilities, relationship of that jobs with other jobs in a concern etc. can be categorized under physical, mental, emotional, social, behavioral specification that can be converted into employee specification.

Advantages

Job specification is useful in:

- Furnishing the requirements of employer to the applicants
- Recruiting an appropriate person for an appropriate position
- Screening
- Give due justification to each job
- Designing training and development programs
- Counseling and monitoring performance of employees
- Job evaluation
- Taking decision by the management regarding promotions, transfers and giving extra benefit to the nurses.

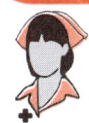

Characteristics

Job specification must specify:

- Nature and functions of the job and the role of the candidate in the particular position
- The educational qualification needed for the job
- The responsibility and accountability of the job position
- Salary structure.

Design

The job specification should have a definite way of writing. It should be objective and to the point and should convey the requirement process. The following items should be included in chronological order:

- The job title
- Reporting to
- A brief overview of nature of the job
- A brief about traits, personality of a candidate requires for the post
- Description the duties and responsibilities a candidate should possess
- Details of the qualification, experience and other specific vocational attributes related to the position
- Overview of the skill and abilities of an applicant for the post
- Description of physical attributes it essential for the job
- Work timings, hours and details of the work environment
- Details of the remunerations and the payment.

STAFF DEVELOPMENT AND STAFF WELFARE

Staff development is the process through which professional growth of employees take place. After sometime, these employees/workers need more skills to tackle the situation as demand increases. Fast technology/advance technology, is the main cause to improve skills to achieve the organizational goals. There is a dire need to change the attitude, knowledge and skills of the vested employees. Staff development is a broader concept whereas inservice education is a narrow concept. Staff development is needed for future needs. Staff development includes both formal and informal activities related to employees within or outside the organization.

Definition

Staff development refers to the processes, programs and activities through which every organization develops, enhances and improves the skills, competences and overall performance of its employees and workers.

Staff development includes all planned education, activities recognized by a health care agency as directed towards meeting the job related learning need of the nurse and other personnel.

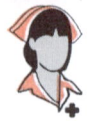

Need of Staff Development Program

- **Social change:** Staff development is of great need due to rapid, social change within past two decades. Influences marked changes in demographic characteristics of population.
- **Scientific advancement:** This is an increased public interest in health promotion, increased technical skills and all new researches in medical, nursing and other health related fields has become the need of the hour.
- **Opportunity for nurses:** All the three basic nursing education programs provide the beginning practitioner with basis understanding and skills upon which the graduate nurse must build a super structure of specific job knowledge and skill in order to meet job requirement.

Goals

- Assist each employee (nurse) to improve performance in his/her position
- Assist each employee to acquire personal and professional abilities that maximize the possibility of career advancement.

Objectives

- To increase employee productivity
- To ensure satisfactory job performance by health personnel
- To ensure safe and effective patient care by nurses
- It helps the personal ensures thinking on job, reduces mechanical action to a minimum and promotes economy, safely and efficiency of personal in their work situation
- To discover potentialities, to alert personalities, to alert personnel in working environment
- Helps to fill the gap between the practice and theory and the utilities of the new researches in nursing.

Resources

There are so many resources which help in development progress are:
- Public libraries
- Audiovisual programs
- Computers
- Different schools and universities
- Open universities
- Associations and health service agencies
- Own staff and other nursing homes.

Guidelines

- Set the physical layout with equipment for the study or work
- Create learning environment
- Explain the ideology and the other factors of the study
- If it is demonstration, do step-by-step

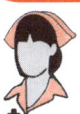

- Have the effective return demonstration in case of practicals.
- Arrange for follow-up.

Process (Flow Chart 9)

Flow Chart 9: Process of staff development

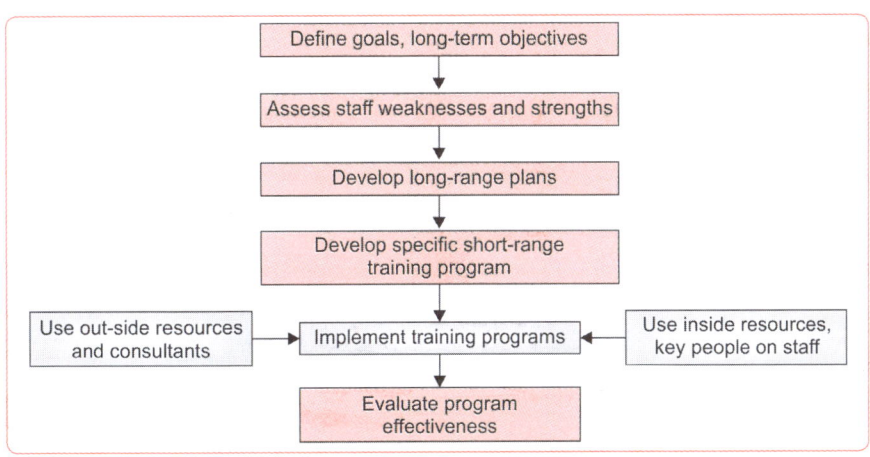

Types

Staff development includes all training and education undertaken by an employer to improve the occupational and personal knowledge, skill and attitude of nurses. The goal of staff development is to assist the individual worker towards clinical improvement personal advancement, and occupational progress. Staff development activities include:

- Induction training
- Job orientation
- Inservice education
- Continuing education
- Training for special function.

Features

The main features of the staff development are:

- Staff development is a broader concept
- Staff development is for future need
- Staff development takes place within or outside the organization
- Staff development includes formal and informal activities related to employees
- It should help the employees in learning and improve knowledge, skill and attitude.

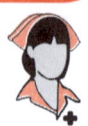

Benefits

- ❏ It benefits the organization and keeps the nursing staff enthusiastic in their learning
- ❏ Job satisfaction among employees
- ❏ Create opportunities for growth and communication
- ❏ Develops sense of responsibility among employees
- ❏ Helps the employees to adjust according to need
- ❏ Helps in developing skills like public relation, interpersonal and human relation skills
- ❏ Helps in making sound decisions.

Benefits to Individual

- ❏ Leads to improve professional practice
- ❏ Aids in updating skills and knowledge
- ❏ Helps the employees to maintain old competencies
- ❏ Helps in adept to change.

STAFF WELFARE

The conditions under which the teaching staff have an effect on the implementation of program besides contributing towards the stability of the staff. Frustration, conflicts, resignations and frequent requesting for transfer can often be reduced when there are clearly defined policies related to hours of work, teaching load, welfare of staff and other matters.

The policies should be written down known to everyone. The following are some of these matters:

Hours of Work

This policy should give clear direction on:
- ❏ Maximum number of hours to be worked per week
- ❏ Number of days off per month
- ❏ Procedure to be followed regarding public holidays
- ❏ Hours to be work for evening or night shift.

Teaching Load

How much a teacher can take load for teaching the students?
- ❏ Time for preparation of class and laboratory classes
- ❏ Students guidance and counseling
- ❏ Evaluation of student's assignments, tests, texts, etc.
- ❏ Committee work
- ❏ Record keeping
- ❏ 20 hours/week of formal teaching like that the recommended time should not exceed.

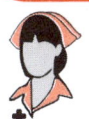

Residence

Staff accommodation for married and single staff with modern facilities should be available to carry out the students curricular or extracurricular activities.

Leave

The institution should have a clear policy regarding:

❑   Like casual leave policy
❑   Provision for maternity leave
❑   How much leave may be taken at a time
❑   Time of year during which annual leave may normally be taken.

Sickness

The policy should include:

❑   Who will be responsible for medical treatment
❑   In parent hospital kind of accommodation which will be given—private, semiprivate or general ward.
❑   The financial responsibility to be borne by the staff member.

Attendance

A conferences and study courses policies regarding selection and deputation of the staff for further education, including attendance at formal courses, refresher courses, workshops, and conferences.

This may depend upon the:

❑   Educational qualification
❑   Years of experience
❑   Any required period of work after return from study
❑   Rotation of staff and number who may attend at one time
❑   Periodic compulsory refresher courses for particular grades of staff.

Continuing education and inservice education:

❑   Employment
     ■   Uniformity in procedure
     ■   Recruitment according to education and experience
❑   Job description
❑   Working hours
❑   Work load facilities
❑   Pay and allowances

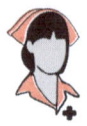

- ❑ Promotional opportunities
- ❑ Career development
- ❑ Accommodation
- ❑ Transport facilities.

DIRECTING

It is the main function of the management process. The foundation provided through planning, shape given by organizing, life installed by staffing are followed by directing which sustains the life of organization, in that it give guidance and directives to the members of organization. Directing entails guiding and supervising personnel to bring about purposeful action towards the desired objective. Directing in the means through which managerial decisions are translated into concentrate action.

Definitions

Directing is the interpersonal aspect of managing by which subordinates are led to understand and contribute effectively and attainment of enterprise objectives.   —*Koontz and O'Donnell*

Directing and telling people what to do and seeing that they do it to the best of their ability. It includes making assignments corresponding procedures, seeing that mistakes are corrected, providing on the job instruction and of course issuing orders.   —*Ernest Dale*

Nature and Features

- ❑ Maintenance of linkage in the various activities performed by various people.
- ❑ Concentration on performance of individual members and group performance.
- ❑ Dealing with human beings has different human factors.
- ❑ Close connection with organization, staffing and coordination function.

Directing includes these sub-functions:

- ❑ **Communication:** It is the process through which manage or instruction/follow-up action/submission of data, etc. is passed on from individual to manager, supervisor and vice versa. Improper or gap in communication leads to mismanagement and maladministration.
- ❑ **Leadership:** A good leader of a team takes the team to the highest peak. Leadership qualities demand the manager to set an example in all respects before the subordinates who normally tend to emulate the leader. Hence a good and effective leadership is essential to provide better administration.
- ❑ **Motivation:** Motivation is must to enhance the interest to work among the workers. A good worker can be motivated to become better and best worker. Motivation depends upon various needs of the person, viz. physiological, safety, social, self-esteem and self-actualization need are required to be fulfilled by the administration. Motivation thus assumes tremendous importance for effective and efficient administration.

Direction is also involved with:

- ❑ Training and instructing subordinates in carrying out their assigned responsibility in the job situation.
- ❑ Motivating the organizational members to meet the expectations of the top management in realizing the goals of the organization.

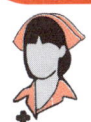

CONTROL—QUALITY MANAGEMENT

Quality control is a specific type of controlling which refers to activities that can evaluate and request the services which are rendered to the consumers. In nursing, the goal of quality care is ensured while meeting intended goals.

Quality Control as Process

The process when viewed simplistically can be broken down into three basic steps:

- The criteria or standard is determined
- Information is collected to determine if standards have been met
- Educational or corrective action is taken if the criteria have not been met.

Total Quality Management/Continuous Quality Improvement

Total quality management (TQM), also referred to as continuous quality improvement (CQI) is based on the premise that the individual is focal element on which production and service depend. Quality is built into the service or product, rather than assuming that inspection of and removal of errors lead to quality. The ultimate responsibility for TQM belongs to top level management, cooperation and support must filter from top of the organization hierarchy down to subordinates.

Principles

Total quality management has the aim to deliver the perfect quality products to the consumers. It has the following principles:

- **Executive management:** Top management mainly creates the environment for quality products.
- **Training:** Training to the new employees or the development programs for the old employees helps in quality management.
- **Customer focus:** The satisfaction of the customer should be the bench mark for the quality.
- **Continuous improvement:** The improvement should not be static, it should be a continuous process.
- **Company culture:** Work culture which promotes the quality should be inculcated in the organization.
- **Employee involvement:** Employees should be encouraged to address the problems related to quality.

The quality assurance activities in the hospital are:

- Nursing care adult
- Direct observation
- Review of documents
- Patients/attendants questionnaire or interviews
- Review of complaints
- Staff questionnaire/interview
- Post-care staff conferences
- Statistical information regarding indicators/checklists.
- Measurement of the nursing competencies

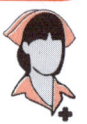

❏ Equipment, e.g. sound level meters.
❏ Peer review
❏ Patient's opinion studies.

BUDGET

Administration may be defined as all actions rationally performed by one person or a number of persons in concert to fulfill a common purpose set by someone else of their accomplishment.

Meaning

Literally the word budget means a leather bag to carry official papers in. This word is derived from the old English word "budgettee" which means a sack or pouch. Budget is the heart of administrative management. It is a formal expression of policies, plan, objectives and goals laid down in advance by top level authorities of the organization as a whole in a given period of time.

Definitions

❏ Budget is a concrete precise picture of the total operation of an enterprise in monetary terms.
—*HM Donovan*
❏ Budgeting involves establishing a financial plan for operating a unit, department and organization.
❏ Budget is an operational plan for a definite period, usually a year, expressed in financial terms and based on expected income and expenditure.

Nursing budget: A plan for allocation of resources based preconceived needs for a proposed series of programs to deliver patient care during one fiscal year.

Principles

❏ It should provide sound financial management by focusing on requirement of the organization.
❏ It should focus on objectives and policies of the organization.
❏ It should ensure the most effective use of scarce financial and nonfinancial resources.
❏ Budget requires that a program's activities are planned in advance.
❏ Budgetary process require consistent delegation for which fixed duties and responsibilities are required to be allocated to managers at different level for framing and executing budget.
❏ Budgeting should include coordinating efforts of various departments establishing a frame of reference for managerial decisions and providing a criterion for evaluating managerial performance.
❏ Utmost care is a must for fixing budget targets.
❏ Budget period must be appropriate to the nature of business or service and to the type of budget.
❏ Budget is prepared under the direction and supervision of the administrator or financial officers.
❏ Budgets are to be prepared and interpreted consistently throughout the organization in the communication of planning process.

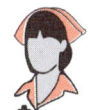

- Budget necessitates a review of the performance of the previous year and an evaluation of its adequacy both in quantity and quality.
- While developing a budget, the provision should be made for its flexibility.

Prerequisites for Budgeting

- Sound organizational structure with clear lines of authority and responsibility is needed.
- Nonmonetary statistical data such as number of admissions, average length of stay, percentage of occupancy and number of patient days—are used for planning and control of the budgetary process.
- Chart of accounts are designed to be consistent with the organization plan.
- Management support is essential for a budgetary program.
- Formal budgeting policies and procedures should be available in the budget manual.
- **Economic goods:** These are goods or services purchased by consumers from suppliers to provide a benefit to the consumers.
- **Income:** Additional resources gained over time
- **Utility:** It is the benefit consumers get from the purchase of goods and services.
- **Marginal utility:** It is the additional utility gained by consuming one more unit
- **Supply:** It is the amount of goods or services the supplier are willing to provide at a given price
- **Demand:** It is the amount of goods or service the consumers are willing to buy at that price
- **Elasticity of demand:** It is the degree to which the demand for a good or service decreases in response to a price increase and increases in response to price decrease
- **Cost factor:** Cost is money expended for all resources used
- **Expenses:** Cost of providing services to patients also called Overhead
- **Expense budgeting:** The process of forecasting recording and monitoring the manpower, materials and suppliers and monetary needs of an organization
- **Types of expense or cost fixed:** They remain constant as volume increase and decreases over a period of time
- **Variable cost:** Relate to volume and census
- **Sunk cost:** Fixed expenses that cannot be recovered even if a program is cancelled
- **Direct cost:** The cost of providing and service
- **Cost accounting:** System assigns all cost to cost centers.

Importance

- Budget is needed for planning for future course of action and to have a control over all the activities in the organization.
- Budget facilities coordinating operation of various department and sections for realizing organizational objectives.
- Budget serves as a guide for action in the organization.
- Budget helps one to weigh the values and to make decision when necessary on whether one is of a greater value in the program than the other.

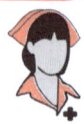

Functions

❑ Budgeting is a complex task; it serves both planning and control functions, which require different orientations to change (Table 2).

Table 2: Functions of budget

S. No.	Planning	Controlling
1.	Requires an expansive or innovative stance	Requires a conservative stance
2.	Early stages of planning focus on general and imprecise goals	Control focuses on specific criteria and comparisons
3.	Forward looking, expansive imprecise	Backward looking, conservative, precise

Classification

Budget consists mainly three sections, i.e. manpower budget, capital expenditure budget, and operating budget:

❑ The *manpower budget* includes wages and other benefits provided for regular and temporary workers.

❑ The *capital expenditure* budget includes purchases of land, buildings, and major equipment of considerable expense and long life that affect operation of more than one unit and commit the agency to a particular course.

❑ The *operating budget* is an agency's financial plan for achieving short range goals over the next 12 months period. It includes the cost of supplies, minor equipment, repair and overheard expenses.

Types

There are several types of budget as follows:

❑ **Incremental budget:** It is based on estimated changes in present operations, plus a percentage increase for inflation, all of which is added to the previous years budget.

❑ **Open ended budget:** It is a financial plan in which each operating manager presents a single cost estimate for it considered optimal activity level for each program in the unit, without indicating how the budget should be scaled down if less funding available.

❑ **Fixed ceiling budget:** It is a financial plan in which the upper most spending limit is set by the top executive before unit and divisional managers develop budget proposals for their areas of responsibility. It forces each manager to relative merits of alternative program.

❑ **Flexible budget:** It is based on the fact that operating conditions rarely conform to expectations. Therefore a flexible budget consists of several financial plans, each for a different level of program activity.

❑ **Roll over budget:** It is one that forecasts program revenues and expenses for period greater than a year, to accommodate program that are longer than the annual budget cycle.

❑ **Performance budget:** It is based on function such as direct nursing care, inservice education, quality improvement and nursing research.

❑ **Program budget:** It is one where costs are computed for a total program, such as ambulatory program.

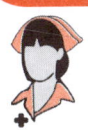

- ❏ **Zero-based budget:** It requires the manager to justify each cost of every program, both old and new, in every annual budget preparation.
- ❏ **Sunset budget:** It is designed to "self-destruct" within a prescribed time period to ensure the cessation of spending by a predetermined date.
- ❏ **Sales budget:** It is the starting point in a budgetary program, since sales are basic activities which give shape to all other activities.
- ❏ **Production budget:** It is the budget that aims at securing the economical manufacture of products and maximizing the utilization of production facilities.
- ❏ **Cash budget:** It is prepared by way of projecting the possible cash receipt and payments over the budget period.
- ❏ **Line item budget:** Itemize workers, machines, supplies by groups. It is primarily a device for controlling expenditures. It used in planning and decision making.

Budgeting Procedure

The budgeting procedure serves both planning and control function. The nurse manager should use a system approach. Designing and implementing a planning program budgeting cycles as follows:

- ❏ Agency goals are reviewed to identify activities of highest priority, because these are most likely to receive funding.
- ❏ Objectives are reviewed for existing programs and written for proposed programs to ensure that achievement of these objectives will support agency mission.
- ❏ Existing programs are revised and proposed program designed to maximize goal achievement.
- ❏ Labor, capital and operating expenses are computed for each program, old and new.
- ❏ Alternative methods are identified for realizing designated objectives and the price of each alternative is determined.
- ❏ Comparisons are made to determine which alternative is most cost-effective.
- ❏ A budget request is developed that details a fiscal plan for the preferred program, indicates alternative methods for meeting the same objectives and explain why the recommended program is preferred.

It is impossible to foresee all events and conditions that can affect the health agency functioning therefore a nurse executive must sometimes submit a supplementary budget item request or proposal at some time other than the regular budget submission period.

Budget Stages

Formulation Stage

- ❏ Usually a set number of months before the start of fiscal year for the budget
- ❏ Develop objectives and management plans
- ❏ Gather all financial, historical, and statistical data and distribute to cost center manager.

Analyze Data

- ❏ Review and enactment
- ❏ Prepare unit budget

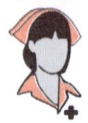

- Present unit budget for approval
- Revise and combine into organizational budget
- Revise and distribute to cost center.

Execution Stage

- Direct and evaluate expenses and receipts
- Revise budget if indicated.

Tools Used in Budget Preparation

Several tools are used in preparing a nursing budget. The most common are work sampling, system sampling, trend analysis, cost benefit analysis and marginal analysis:

Work Sampling

It is an individual engineering technique, in which an individual from outside the primary work group observes the activities of a selected sample of employees at regular intervals, records the activity each is engaged in and generalizes from the observed sample of the worker's activities to estimate the percentage of the employer's total work time spent in each task. More reliable information can be obtained by work sampling than employee self-report because a disinterested outsider will measure time objectively than an employee whose job security may be threatening if study result reveals inefficient time use.

System Analysis

In this a nursing program is viewed as a complex, an interrelated series of steps in which specific input of employees, material and equipment are subjected to designated throughput processes to produce a desired service output. It is helpful in replanning or adjusting an inefficient service program, because step by step examination of a complex process often reveals workable alternatives to malfunctioning system segments. By analyzing the nursing process systematically the manger can discover ways in which to improve patient care by altering the number or type of personnel assigned, rescheduling activities, changing the relationship of patients to personnel, or improving the manger's information about patient census, patient classification, or acuity or staff availability.

Trend Analysis

It is a mathematic tool whereby a manager graphs data from the preceding three to five tears related to the following factors:

- Patient census
- Patient diagnosis
- Patient length of stay
- Staff seniority
- Staff turnover
- Staff sick or absent time
- Hours of care per patient per day delivered by each employee
- Classification and daily cost of direct nursing care per patient per day.

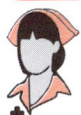

Trend analysis often yields information of value in budget planning. However, factors other than historical trends also influence future nursing supply and demand. Among these are population changes, medical staff characteristics, technological breakthrough, weather changes and alteration in the nation's work or recreational patterns.

Cost Benefit Ratio

It is a numerical relationship between the value of a program's costs and the value of the program's benefits. The cost effective ratio is expressed as a fraction. If the fraction is greater than 1, i.e. if benefits outweigh costs, the program is economically worthwhile. The cost benefit ratio is useful in selecting the best of several alternative programs. Unfortunately the ratio is difficult to compute, because much expenditure are impossible to separate on a program-to-program basis. It is difficult to determine what proportion of the agency's nursing research costs should be charged to each nursing unit. In addition, many program benefits cannot be expressed in financial terms. It is impossible to establish the monetary value of improved moral and self-esteem experienced by patients who are cared for under primary or case methods of nursing are delivery.

Marginal Analysis

It is a mathematical tool by which a manager computers the additional value to

How to Improve Budget Estimate Smart

Here are some specific, measurable, attainable, realistic and tangible top 11 lessons which would help in improving the estimation technique:

1. Institutionalize a culture to educate project teams about estimation (techniques/tools)
2. Encourage use of appropriate estimation techniques for different phases of the project life cycle.
3. Empower project manager to estimate and re-estimate after every phase of the project life cycle (if necessary).
4. Clearly defined guidelines for creating estimate baselines should be in place.
5. Every change request should be documented and estimated.
6. Estimation once done should not be considered as sacrosanct. There should be provision to revise it if the circumstances under which it was prepared for the first time change.
7. Project needs and requirements should be documented in such a way that inputs, outputs and process is defined. The clearer the input, the better is the estimate.
8. Leverage historical information about project's effort, schedule, cost, risk, and resources which can be referred as lessons learned/best practices from engagements executed in the past. Statistical baselines should be created for each factor affecting project effort, e.g. user training effort baseline or project management effort baseline. These statistical baselines should be revised periodically.
9. Propagate the culture to define work packages and track time against them diligently. (Project management tools should be provided to do so.)
10. Every organization has influence on overall project effort which should be considered while estimating the project timelines as each organization has their own tried and tested way of executing project based on their available skill set and capability with the client.

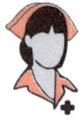

11. One aspect of project estimation which has been ignored most of the time is size estimation which is very essential to measure project performance, build baselines or perform comparative analysis. Organizations should perform size estimate and use organizational productivity baseline (per size unit) for estimating project effort.

Estimation of a Budget for Nursing Services

In preparing a budget for nursing service the income and the expenditure incurred towards nurses and nursing are to be shown. The expenditure will have to reflect:

❑ The amount of money spent towards basic pay and allowances of all categories of nurses employed in the institution per annum.

❑ The amount of money spent towards nurses' welfare activities, pension, provident fund and gratuity if any, per annum.

❑ The expenditure involved towards nursing staff development program during the year under reference.

❑ The expenditure towards extracurricular activities organized by the organization during the period under reference.

Difficulties in Making Budget Estimate

❑ There may not be as much historical data or none at all

❑ Even with similar projects, there may be significant differences

❑ Multiple people have input to the budget

❑ Continued estimating budgets are difficult

❑ Multiple people have some control over the budget

❑ There is more "flexibility" regarding the estimates of inputs (material and labor)

❑ The accounting system may not be set up to track project data

❑ Usage of labor and material is very lumpy over time.

Benefits of Budget Estimate

Some of the major advantages of budget planning are:

❑ It puts checks or balances in place in order to prevent overspending at various levels

❑ Takes into account the unexpected need for funds

❑ Help one maintain his/her standard of living post retirement

❑ Make better investment decisions

❑ Generate more return on investment (ROI)

❑ Gain advantage over competitors by taking appropriate and timely decisions

❑ More control over project execution

❑ Finally improve organizational productivity.

Disadvantages/Risks of Budget Estimate

Budget estimate has the following shortcomings:

❑ Excessive emphasis on savings may affect the quality of life

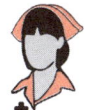

- ❏ If the budget is planned too tight, adherence to it may become an issue
- ❏ Lack of knowledge on how to estimate and estimation techniques
- ❏ Adoption of inappropriate estimation methodologies
- ❏ Misinterpretation of available historical information
- ❏ Lack of information necessary for estimation
- ❏ Inadequate timeframe to perform estimates
- ❏ Insufficient experience in doing estimation for similar kind of work
- ❏ Even with careful planning, estimates are wrong
- ❏ Most firms add 5–10% for contingencies
- ❏ Other bidding factors
  - ▪ Escalation
  - ▪ Waste
  - ▪ Bad luck

Assessing the Soundness of the Budget

The soundness of budget systems can be judged by the following:

Comprehensiveness

- ❏ Is the coverage of government operations complete?
- ❏ Are estimates gross or does netting take place?

Transparency

- ❏ How useful is the budget classification? Are there separate economic and functional classifications that meet international standards?
- ❏ Is it easy to connect policies and expenditures through a program structure?

Realism

- ❏ Is the budget based on a realistic macroeconomic framework?
- ❏ Are estimates based on reasonable revenue projections? How are these made, and by whom?
- ❏ Are the financing provisions realistic?
- ❏ Is there a realistic costing of policies and programs and hence expenditures (e.g. assumptions about inflation, exchange rates, etc.)
- ❏ How are future cost implications taken into account?
- ❏ Is there a clear separation between present and new policies?
- ❏ How far are spending priorities determined and agreed under the budget process?

Revised Estimate

- ❏ In calculating quarterly GDP, a third estimate published approximately three months after the end of a *quarter*. It includes information not available at the time of *advance estimate* or

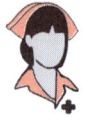

preliminary estimate, as well as any necessary data revisions. However, it is still subject to scrutiny and potential alteration.

❑ A change in the calculation of the cost of a *project*. This calculation is made and presented to a *buyer*, usually while a project is in progress, and may be subject to further changes due to both exogenous factors and endogenous factors.

A revised estimate is based on:

❑ Ascertained actual of the past months of a financial year, and
❑ An estimate of the probable figure for the remaining months of that year.

Reviews

❑ Budget implementation should be reviewed periodically to ensure that program are implemented effectively and to identify and financial or policy slip-ups.
❑ The review of budget execution should cover financial, physical and other performance indicators.
❑ Cost increases due to inflation, unexpected difficulties, insufficient initial study of projects, and budget overruns must be identified so that adequate counter measures can be prepared.
❑ A comprehensive mid-term review of the implementation of the budget is needed, while the financial implementation of the budget should be reviewed monthly.
❑ Development budgets are often beset by implementation problems because of insufficient implementation capacities and other factors such as delays in mobilizing external financing, over optimistic implementation schedules, climatic hazards, or difficulties in importing supplies.
❑ Mechanisms for reviewing the most significant or problematic projects are needed. These could consist of a regular monthly or quarterly.
❑ Review of projects within line ministries and a mid-year review involving lines ministries and center agency.

In-year Budget Revision

❑ It is difficult to make accurate forecast for the implementation of certain programs or for developments in economic parameters such as inflation, interest rate or exchange rates.
❑ Some immediate needs that were not foreseen during budget execution may appear during budget execution.
❑ Limit the effects of these problems, rules for transfers must be flexible appropriations for debt service cannot be a spending limit and should be revised according to developments in interest rates or the exchange rate.
❑ However, their amount must account for only 1–3% of the total budget; otherwise, budget execution will involve bargaining the uses of reserves and the budget will become an allocation of reserves.
❑ Therefore, for changes that after the composition of the budget or when an overall increase in expenditures is unavoidable the budget may have to be revised. Mechanisms for revisions depend on the countries, and should be clearly stated in the budget organic law.

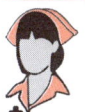

- Some broad principles are desirable. Since the budget has been passed by the legislature, revisions should be made by law.
- Generally, changes in appropriation above a certain percentage of the initial appropriation of changes that affect the total amount of expenditures must be submitted for to the legislature for approval.
- To allow the government to address problems with dispatch, procedures authorizing exceptional expenditures before the Parliament approves them can be considered.
- However, the authority should be regulated and limited, and the executive must be required to present a revised budget to the Parliament at short notice.
- Supplementary estimates should be approved only at a fixed time and the number of in-year revisions should be strictly limited (to preferably only one in-year budget revision).
- Some countries present supplementary estimates to Parliament on a case-to-case basis, each time the Cabinet approves a request from a line ministry be, as a result, an excessive number of supplementary estimates are prepared every year. Such procedures should be avoided.
- Budget execution is difficult to control when budget is continually being revised.
- Budget revision should be made during the fiscal year and requests from line ministries should be reviewed together, not singly.

MANAGEMENT PROCESS

Retaining

An institute can be able to get the best employees ever by a good and efficient recruitment cell. Now the challenge comes, that how to retain them in the institute. The institute should have some strategies to retain the employees in the organization:

- **Selecting and training:** After the selection, organization should take the steps to develop more skills in their employees through training. This helps the employee to adjust and merge in the working culture of the organization.
- **An effective orientation:** It helps the employee to understand the work environment and organization and aids to adjust in the environment.
- **Job satisfaction:** Lower job satisfaction leads to more resignation rate of employees. So the policies should be employee friendly so that person can do the job with satisfaction.
- **Creating trust:** Trust between the employee and employer, management and work team leads to the long journey of the job in the organization.
- **Empower to the employees:** It is essential to empower each employee in the organization irrespective to her level of work in in the organization. Each employ should enjoy the autonomy while doing the job.
- **Recognize employees:** Prioritize the recognition of each personnel and help them to retain in the organization.
- **Stress management:** Dissatisfaction, boredom leads to the stress. Attention should be given on innovation, special career needs, determining their other needs and help at time. All these things manages to stress management.

    These all help in retaining the employee in the organization.

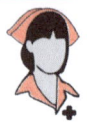

Superannuation

Superannuation is an organizational pension program created by a company for the benefits of its employee. Pension is the money which the employee get after the retirement. It also refers as company pension plan. The funds which are deposited in a superannuation account will grow typically without any tax implications until retirement or withdrawal of money.

It can be:

❑ Employee provident fund (EPF)

❑ Public provident fund (PPF)

❑ National pension scheme (NPS) etc.

The main advantage of superannuation fund is that the employee can set up a regular savings program and make lump-sum payments. Employee's resources are pooled with other inverters, allowing them to make investments impossible for an individual investor. It helps the employee to easily diversify his /her investments.

Coordination and Control

Coordination is the process of balancing and keeping the team together by ensuring a suitable allocation of working activities to the various members, and seeing that these are performed with due harmony among the members themselves.

The need of coordination arises due to some of the following factors in the organization. They are:

❑ Diverse and specialized activities

❑ Empire building

❑ Personal rivalries and prejudice

❑ Conflict of interest

The main importance of coordination is

❑ With the coordination only, the team spirit can arise and the coordination of all efforts, forces and activities within and without, help to achieve the goals of organization.

❑ It leads to group efforts which have always more impact than individual.

❑ It helps to get the unity of direction by way of securing spontaneous collaboration on the part of different departments.

❑ It helps to tones up the general level of employees morale and provides job satisfaction.

There are certain techniques of coordination which helps to start, and maintain the coordination in a positive way so that the coordination helps to achieve the organizational goals. The techniques are:

❑ Good communication, on the other hand no communication gaps

❑ Policies, procedures, and standing orders should be orderly planned

❑ Effective supervision

❑ Motivational leadership

❑ Interaction and correlation within and interdepartments should be encouraged.

❑ Direct contact with management members to exchange ideas and view-points.

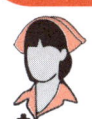

CONTROL

Control ensures the realization of planned objectives through the process of work evaluation. The Work progress is analyzed and appraised in terms of quality, quantity time use and cost.

In other words control in to see how far coordination has become effective in the organization. If any deficiency is found, corrective actions are taken to bring back needed coordination into full play for putting the performance on proper track.

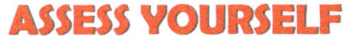

ASSESS YOURSELF

1. Explain management process in details.
2. As a head nurse how will you recruit staff nurses for ten bedded ICU unit in your hospital.
3. Explain the role of head nurse in budget making.

Physical Layout of Hospital

Learning Objective

☞ Explain the administration of different health care units.

Key Terms

⊷ **Hospital:** Social and medical organization for health care.

⊷ **Therapeutic environment:** Environment which helps in early healing.

⊷ **Esthetics:** Beauty (physical)

⊷ **Nosocomial infection:** Hospital acquired infection.

Before learning the physical layout of hospital we should know what a hospital is? According to WHO, "A hospital is an integral part of a social and medical organization, the function of which is to maintain the complete health care, both curative and preventive and whose outpatient service reach out to the family and its home environment". In fact hospital is an institution suitably located, constructed, organized, staffed to supply scientifically, economically efficiently and unhindered health care and treatment by specialized staff and equipment.

Modern hospitals are classified as according to following criteria:

❑ Length of stay of patient: (Long-term and short-term)

❑ Clinical basis

❑ Ownership/control basis

❑ Objective basis

❑ Size basis

❑ Management

❑ System of medicine basis

The main functions of the hospital are:

❑ Patient care

❑ Diagnosis and treatment of the disease

❑ Outpatient services

❑ Medical education and training

❑ Medical and nursing research

❑ Prevention of disease and promotion of health.

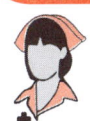

PHYSICAL LAYOUT

Physical layout of the hospital helps to create the comfort to the caretakers and caregivers. It increases the efficiency of the whole system by decreasing the unnecessary botherations and contamination. The physical layout attracts the clients especially in the private hospitals so the emphasis is done on physical layout.

Efficiency and Cost Effectiveness

An efficient hospital layout should:
- Frequently used spaces should have minimum distance.
- Staff should have easy visual supervision of patients by constructing recovery rooms.
- Only required areas should be constructed.
- Provide an efficient logistics systems including elevators, in-built tubes, good arrangements for food process, clean supplies and removal of waste, recyclables, etc.
- Space should be utilized properly by combining the requirements and make prudent use of multipurpose spaces.
- The places should be according to the need of care givers and caretakers.

Flexibility and Expandability

As the medical needs changes day-by-day but we cannot change the physical constructions day-by-day so these should be so constructed that with the planning the changes can be made easily. It should have a flexible and easily modified mechanical and electrical system. Size should be so that the changes in the wards or areas can be made possible. Renovation should be easy. There should be space for the expandability if needed. It should be an open ended, well planned in all directions for future expansion.

Therapeutic Environment

Therapeutic environment helps the patient to feel comfortable even in dim situation. Hospital infection, also called nosocomial infection halts the therapeutic environment. With the interior design we can create the therapeutic environment by understanding the patient's profile and the work of the care givers. Some important aspects of creating therapeutic environment according to physical layout may be as follows:
- Culturally relevant material which consists with sanitation and functional needs should be used.
- Avoid the colors which can irritate the patients or can cause the interference with diagnosis, e.g. yellow color in neonatal nursing.
- Sunlight should enter in each corner of the hospital. It is a natural disinfectant.
- Big windows should be there, as the natural scenes have also a healing power. If not possible big natural pictures should be placed.
- Designing should be such which helps the patients or their relative to move safe and easy from one place to another place.

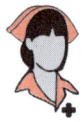

Cleanliness and Sanitation

Hospitals must be easy to clean and maintain. This is facilitated by:

❏ Appropriate, durable finishes for each functional space.

❏ Careful detailing of such features as door frames, case work and finish transitions to avoid dirt catching and hard to clean services and joints

❏ Adequately and appropriately located housekeeping spaces.

❏ Special materials, finishes and details for spaces which are to be kept sterile, such as integral cove base. The new antimicrobial surfaces might be considered for appropriate locations.

❏ Stress should be taken for indoor environmental quality.

❏ Wash up area, laundry area, scrubbing area, etc. should be of easy to maintain type.

Accessibility

Accessibility to the hospital to all areas including both inside and outside should have complied with minimum requirements and should be designed easy to be used by the patient's especially handicapped or orthopedic patients and their relatives. Gardens, corridors, stairs should be enough specious for the use of the caretakers. Glow marks from the entrance to the different area or the other prominent indicators should be there.

Controlled Circulation

Hospitals are always having a complex system of interrelated functions which require the movement of the people and goods. These circulations can be the source of infection so it should be controlled.

❏ Outpatients department should be away from the wards or it should be separate from inpatient area.

❏ Route and ways for outpatient should be properly marked.

❏ The nursing personnel or caregiver should have a separate way to reach.

❏ Separate type of patients should be on separate areas.

❏ Mortuary and the way to mortuary should be from the back door.

❏ Trash, social material should also move from back door.

❏ Good and safe elevators should be available for the heavy and other goods.

❏ Emergency area should be at one side of the hospital.

Esthetics

As we already read that for therapeutic environment esthetics has big role. Nowadays the concentration on the aesthetics of the hospitals is in fashion. Increased use of natural light like making domes, etc. natural material like having plants inside the buildings is common. The use of art work, good furniture, beautiful color scales, e.g. bright colors with cartoons in pediatric wards are used. The compatibility is used according to physical surroundings.

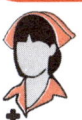

Security and Safety

In addition to safety to the patients in hospital, the security is also an important concern.

- ❑ Protection of drugs and to save misuse of drugs.
- ❑ Control for violence.
- ❑ Security for hospital property and assets.
- ❑ Security against any terrorism act.
- ❑ Safety of physically challenged patients.
- ❑ Safety and security of the working personnel in the hospital.

Sustainability

Hospitals have a sustainable design as it require large amount of energy, water and generates a good amount of waste. These are large buildings so having great sustainability.

Safety Measures for Prevention of Accidents and Infections

An accident has been defined as "an unexpected, unplanned occurrence which may involve injury." According to WHO advisory group "Accident is an unpremeditated event resulting in recognizable damage".

People coming in hospital may be sick, their relatives, and workers. They are both depressed and stressed or in hurry due to tension on the mind. So there are ample causes and reasons for the hospital accidents. By some more measures of safety we may able to prevent the accidents.

Major and various measures can be comprised as follows:

- ❑ **Data collection:** There should be a basic reporting system of all accident so that we can presume where the most accident happens and why this happens? That area should be checked and try to eliminate the cause.
- ❑ **Safety education:** Safety education should be given to the workers and users of the hospital time to time.

Promotion of Safety Measures

Promotion of safety measures like:

- ❑ Maintenance and repair of the buildings
- ❑ Maintenance and repair of the equipment
- ❑ Proper height of walls and parapets
- ❑ Maintenance of the electrical circuits, heaters, air conditioners refrigerators, etc.
- ❑ Proper designs of the building as the parking should be away from the OPDs etc.
- ❑ Alcohol and other drugs should be banned to use in or around hospital premises.
- ❑ Enforcement of law should be done to protect the people from accidents.

Prevention of Infection in Hospitals

Hospital infection is also called nosocomial infection and it affects both patient as well as hospital. In fact patient's immune system may already got weekend from the disease or therapy and hospital

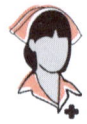

is one of the most likely place for acquiring an infection because of harboring a high population of virulents strains of microorganisms that are usually resistant to antibiotics.

❑ The main aim of the hospital infection control program is to lower the risk of an infection control program in the hospitals which includes:

- An effective system should operate for the surveillance of the risk of hospital infection
- A number of policies should be made to prevent hospital infection
- In service education, seminars, etc. should be conducted time to time about nosocomial infection and its prevention
- Records and reports on the infection should be strictly maintained.

The best way to carry out infection control program in the hospital is to establish and maintain an infection control committee.

The infection control committee should be handed by the hospital administration as infection control officer should have members or committee consisted of representatives of various clinical areas including nursing staff and other heads of all departments of the hospital. The role and responsibility of the infection control committee are as follows:

❑ Information about the infection in detail should be given.

❑ Criteria should be inculcated for reporting the infections.

❑ Reviews of clusters and infected areas should be done.

❑ Proposals and protocols from the hospitals should be approved.

❑ Proper sterilization should be done.

❑ Cleaning agents, their use, their strength, etc. should be checked.

❑ Proper aseptic technique should be used and supervised.

❑ Needed immunization in high risk areas should be provided.

❑ Proper checkups for the food handlers should be there. Infection control officer should have a dedicated team to work day and night, followed by the staff nurses and the supervisors. The table of the infection control nurse will include the following:

- She should visit daily to the assigned wards
- Visitors report register should be checked for the number of visitors
- Daily data of incidence of hospital infection should be recorded
- Hospital infection controls infection should be done in each ward
- Complications of ward wise, discipline wise or procedure wise statistics
- Daily visit to laboratory to ascertain results of previous day sample
- Monitoring and supervision of infection among hospital staff
- Training of nursing aids and paramedical on correct use of hygiene practices and aseptic techniques
- Assist in bacteriological studies in all cases.

Nurses working in intensive care units (ICU) should be particularly conscious of aseptic practice because these patients are already at risk for infection due to so many reasons.

Some good practices of aseptic techniques are as follows:

❑ Segregation of contaminated instruments

❑ Good disinfection practices

❑ Good sterilization practices

❑ Adequate isolation facilities

❑ Maintain antibiotic policy

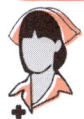

- Taking precautionary measures against cholera, hepatitis, AIDS, etc.
- Good and clean environment at outpatient department (OPD)
- Good dietary services
- Careful handling of soiled linen
- Good housekeeping
- Terminal disinfection of isolation rooms
- Air hygiene of operation theater.
- Developing a sense of awareness in hospital personnel.

There are some universal precautions used by health workers including nurses when caring for all patients also helps infection control.

- Gloves protect the patient as well as care given in the case of in contact with blood, body fluid, open skin lesions or mucus membrane.
- Goggles, masks and face shields, are the weapons to protect from the risk of droplet infections.
- The caregiver should protect herself from needle stick injury etc.

LEGAL RESPONSIBILITIES OF A NURSE

The nurse should be aware of some legal aspects of nursing, e.g. carelessness or negligence. Because of this on the part of the nurse may lead court action against her or hospital. So the knowledge of law about nursing should be known to every nurse for the following two reasons.

1. To protect herself from liability.
2. To ensure the work according to the law.

- **Responsibility in appointing and assigning:** The nurse administrable has responsibility for staffing and supervision nursing units to ensure safe, effective patient care. The manager is also obliged to adjust the amount and type of supervision to fit and employee's level of maturity and experiences.
- **Responsibility in quality control:** A nurse manager legal responsibility for quality control is to observe report and correct the incompetence of any patient care provider. Head nurse is responsible for quality of patient care given by personnel, including medical on the nursing unit.
- **Responsibility for equipment:** A nurse manager must ensure that all the patient care equipment are fully functional and defective equipment are repaired. Storage of patient care equipment is also the responsibility of the nurse. She can also refuse to use the equipment known to be faulty.
- **Responsibility for observing and reporting:** Nursing personnel have more prolonged patient contact. It is the legal duty to observe patient, frequently and report findings infants, children, aged, psychiatric and critically ill patients require keen observation. The nurse has duty to inform about the patient's condition promptly so that physician can base treatment.
- **Responsibility to protect public:** It is a legal duty to protect the public from injury by dangerous patients. The manger must ensure that nursing personnel follow the procedures to alert community to the presence of dangerous patient in their midst.
- **Responsibility for record keeping:** The medical record is essential to proper care. Failure to record significant patient information makes a nurse guilty of negligence. Medical record must be accurate to provide a sound basis for care planning.

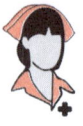

❑ **Responsibility in death and dying:** Nurses must be aware of legal definition of death because they must document all events that when the patient is in their care. Nurse must treat deceased person with dignity and obtaining consent for an autopsy.

LEADERSHIP STYLES

Leadership styles are defined as different combinations of tasks and relationship behaviors used to influence others to accomplish goals (Huber 2000).

Leadership style is the way of providing direction implementing plans and motivating people. It is one of the most important functions of executive to set the direction, to meet the basic goals for organization.

Leaders have to adopt a style, which fits into their subordinate personalities as well as the tasks in hand to achieve maximum effectiveness and efficiency. Leaders have to adopt the leadership style according to the situation. Leadership style and effectiveness of interaction between leadership and their subordinates are important determinants of team success in any hierarchical organization.

Type of Leadership Styles

Several leadership styles have been described:
❑ Charismatic leadership
❑ Authoritarian or directive leadership
❑ Democratic or participative leadership
❑ Laissez-faire or non-directional leadership
❑ Situational leadership
❑ Transactional leadership
❑ Transformational leadership

Three major types of leadership styles are given below:
1. Authoritarian or autocratic leadership
2. Participative or democratic
3. Free-rein or delegative.

Authoritarian Leadership Style

In this style leader is boss. It dictates the policies and procedures and decides what goals are to be achieved and directs and controls all activities without any meaningful participation by the subordinates. In this type of leadership, leaders believe in force.

Dictionary, authoritarian leadership is characterized by an insistence obedience to authority.

In this type of leadership, the leader or authoritarian manager arranges the physical layout so that people cannot form the social group. The employees work in the same way as they were told to do and possible changes or improvements are not tolerated. The psychological need of employees is not considered. The mutual trust is virtually eliminated in such type of leadership. The maximum productivity is achieved by making the worker completely subject to management's dictation.

According to some people, this style is a cruel type style in which the force and unprofessionalism is used to bossing the people around.

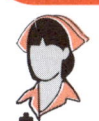

Participative or Democratic Leadership Style

This type of leadership style a participative leader, rather than taking autocratic decisions, seeks to involve other people in the process possibly including subordinates peers, superiors and other stake holders. There are varieties of stages on spectrum depending upon the involvement of people in decision making improves the understanding of issues. People are more committed to action when involved in decision making. This decision making creates a feeling of social commitment to one another.

It involves the leader and team members in making decision. This type of leadership style have benefit for the leader and team as it allows the leader to take decision and the team to have a feeling of part of group of decision making.

Participative Style of Leadership

Democratic leaders offer guidance to group members. In Lewin's study, children in participative leadership style were less productive than members of the authoritarian group, but their contribution were of much higher quality. Group members are more motivated and creative, when involved in decision making process.

Delegative (Free-rein) Leadership Style

This type of leadership style is also known as Laissez-faire. The leader allows the employees are able to analyze the situation and determine what need to be done and how to be done. The leader must have trust and confidence in the employees.

The word Laissez-faire means the noninterference in the affairs of others. It means the leader does not interfere in the decisions of employees in his/her absence. Such type of leaders offers little or no guidance to group members. It is effective in situations where group members are highly qualified in the area of expertise.

There are some other types of leadership also which we have enlisted earlier also.

Participative Leadership Style

The leader involves the employees in taking decision due to which the employees that are more committed to action. It is believed that several people deciding together make decision better than one person along.

Charismatic Leadership Style

There is not any form of external power or authority, by which the leader gathers the followers, but they are gathered through dint of personality and charm. The charismatic leaders have their action words to suit the situation. They engenders trust through visible self-sacrifice and take personal risks in the name of beliefs. They make use of their body language. According to Conger Kanungo (1998) there are five behavioral attributes of charismatic leaders as givens below:

1. Vision and articulation
2. Sensitivity to environment
3. Sensitivity to member needs
4. Personal risk taking
5. Performing unconventional behavior

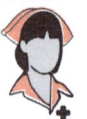

The charismatic leaders are more concerned with themselves. They can have positive or negative impact. Positive effect will occur when they are well intentioned toward others and will elevate and transfer the entire company. The selfish nature will result negative effect and creation of cults. Sometimes, the self-belief can also lead them into psychotic narcissism.

Situational Leadership Style

The decision taken by a leader is not same in every type of situation, i.e. not adopt a single style in each situation, their decision differs according to the need of situations. There are a wide range of factors which influence the decision such as:

- ❑ Motivation and capability of followers
- ❑ Relationship between followers and leader
- ❑ Leader's perception of himself
- ❑ Stress and mood of leader and employee.

Transactional Leadership Style

Transactional leadership is based on reward and punishment. The transactional leaders create a clear structure of what is required from their subordinates and also the reward they get for following orders. When the work is allocated to workers by transactional leaders, they are fully responsible. On success they get rewards and on failure, they got punishment. They use management by exception principle which is that something is operating to defined, performance, than it does not need attention.

Transformational Leadership Style

The transformational leaders put passion and energy into everything and care about employee and encourage them to succeed. It means they get things done by creating enthusiasm and energy among them. These leaders take every opportunity and will use whatever works to convince others to climb the stair of success.

Transformational leader seeks to transform the organization. Transformational are charismatic but are not narcissistic as pure charismatic leaders, who believe in themselves.

Difference between the three types of leadership style is depicted in Table 1.

Table 1: Difference between the main three types of leadership style

Character	Autocratic	Participative	Laissez-faire
Decision making	Employees not involved only leader takes decision	Employees and leader collectively takes decision	Employees take decision but leader is still responsible
Situations where to use	When leader have short of time and is having all information	When leader have part of information and employees have other part of information	When employees are able to analyze the situation and able to determine the needs
Motivation	Less motivated employees	Motivated as involved in decision making	Motivated as free to take decision

contd...

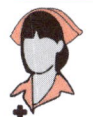

Character	Autocratic	Participative	Laissez-faire
Task delegation	Not	Not	Certain tasks are delegated
Interference	Full interference by leader as he is bossing people around	Interference from both parts, i.e. employees and leader	No interference by leader
Productive	Highly productive	Less productive	Less productive than other two types

PROBLEM SOLVING

Problem solving is a scientific, systematic approach to solve the problem. It involves creative ideas so problem solving is a proven of taking corrective action in order to meet objectives. It is a core function of management. Decision making and problem solving are almost synonymous, both terms can be used interchangeably.

Problems are of many types depending upon the nature, level and process. Some problems can be of serious nature and other can be of routine. These problems may be structural, unstructured, complex, simple, major, minor, etc.

Some examples of problems are as follows:

- Serious or trivial
- Familiar or novel
- Related to work process
- Interpersonal relation
- Related to own level of responsibility
- Related to subordinate level
- Related to supervisor level

Nature and Characteristics

Problem solving is an intellectual activity that involves judgment evaluation and selection. The following are the characteristics of problem solving.

- It has process concept
- Time sequence
- Action commitment
- Evaluation
- Rationality

Principles

Following are the principles that a nurse manager should keep in mind while solving the problem:

- Ensure prompt attention
- Separate large to resolve smaller problems
- Follow policies to resolve smaller problems

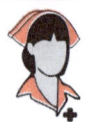

- ❏ Delegate smaller problems to subordinate
- ❏ Consult with management for major problem
- ❏ Consult with experts
- ❏ Relaxed in approaching problem
- ❏ Accept the problem

Problem Solving Approach

Various sequential steps are to be taken to solve the problem:

- ❏ **Tackle problem in sequence:** Take each problem before understanding.
- ❏ **Rank the problem** and handle one at one time in order of priority.
- ❏ **Group the problems:** Group the identified problems on the basis of diagnostic and search activities.

Main Steps of Problem Solving

- ❏ **Step I: Identifying, developing and stating the problem**
  - Select the problem by setting the priority ranking in order.
  - Develop and state problem selected in a precise form.
- ❏ **Step II: Problem analysis and establish solution**
  - Identify the specific problem and diagnose the factors that result in the problem and cause of problem.
  - Data needs to be processed may require collection classification and analysis. Sound decisions are based upon proper collection, classification and analysis of facts and figures. There are three important principles of analysis and classification:
  1. Futurity of the decision (i.e. to what extent of time does the decision commit the work/ business to a course of action)
  2. The impact of decision on the other areas and functions.
  3. The qualitative considerations which come into picture.
     The purpose of classification is to ensure that the decision made takes a comprehensive view of the business as a whole rather than immediate or local problem.
- ❏ **Step III: Developing and finding out alternative solutions:** After analyzing and classifying the problem, the manager has to develop few alternative solutions to solve the problem. The main aim of finding the alternative solutions is to have the best possible decision out of the available alternate course of action. Hypothetical solutions can be established. Techniques like computer appliances, etc. can be helpful for this step.
- ❏ **Step IV: Selecting the best solution/alternative:** After developing so many alternatives now it is a time to see, evaluate and think for the best solution/alternative. While selecting the best solution following factors should be considered:
  - Availability of resources, cost, manpower and methods.
  - Optimum results and consequences.
  - Time consumed.
  - Take a positive attitude towards solution.
- ❏ **Step V: Implementation of the best alternative:** At this step, the manager has to convert the decision into the effective action. For effective execution of the decision it is very important to communicate the decision to the subordinates. The decision should be acceptable to the

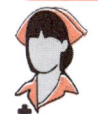

subordinates so as to encourage their involvement. Correct timing of execution of decision minimizes the resistance to change therefore; implementation time also plays a vital role in the proper execution of decision.

❑ **Step VI: Evaluation, feedback and follow-up:** After implementing the best alternative the manager must seek the feedback regarding the effectiveness of the implemented solutions. Feedback allows the manager to become aware of the recent problems associated with the solution. It helps in monitoring the effect of their acts to gauge their success. The evaluation helps to decide the change or continue the same further.

RECORDS AND REPORTS

Records

Record is the permanent written communication that documents information role to a client's health management. "Record" means documents facilitates evaluation of the program and provides continuity from the time the institution is established.

Record is clinical, scientific, administrative legal document relating to the nursing care given to individual, family and community.

Uses

❑ Effective means of communication
❑ Legal documents
❑ Save efforts and money
❑ Help in providing best possible service to the individual, family and community
  ■ Health worker can organize his work and make the most effective use of his time
  ■ Can be useful as an instrument of health education.

Essential Requirements

❑ It should be complete in detail
❑ It should be accurate
❑ Written in such a way that the minimum of clerical work is involved
❑ It should be kept confidential. They should not be shown or discussed with persons other than those providing the health care
❑ Safe keeping of records is must and should be protected against loss.

Cumulative or Continuing Records

Cumulative records have information gathered over a period of time in respect of each patient in different situations. When completed the cumulative records reveals the whole health history of the person.

Design

There are three designs of records:

1. **File type:** For each patient a file is maintained. The outer cover of the file is usually printed with columns for summarizing information. The periodical data are entered in separate leaves of paper and inserted into file.

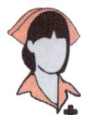

2. **Envelope type:** The file type when closed on three sides and kept open on one will form an envelope. The data are entered on separate level, tagged together and inserted into the envelope.

3. **Folder type:** It is broad card which can be folded into many parts, 8 or 10 pages. Some pages may be kept blank for future entries.

Types

- Village records
- Eligible couple records
- Family folders
- Communicable disease
- Maternal and child health records
- Immunization records
- School health records
- Birth and death records
- Hospital records
- Outdoor attendance register
- Operation register
- Records of medical care
- Daily dairy
- Monthly reports
- Stock registers
- Indoor registers
- Clinical experience records
- Health records
- Periodic evaluation records
- Job descriptions, etc.

Reports

Reports are the subjective written accounts founded upon observant one made by the individuals, who are relating the communications.

Or

Reports are oral or written exchange of information shared between nurses or a number of persons. Report is concise and contains pertinent information. Reporting is the communication of information to another individual.

Purposes

- To show the kind and amount of service rendered over specific period.
- To illustrate progress in reaching goals.
- As an aid in studying health conditions.
- As an aid in planning.

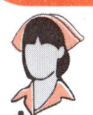

- ❏ To interpret the services to the public and to the other interested agencies.
- ❏ It helps to coordinate care given by several people.
- ❏ It prevents the clients from having to repeat information to each health team members.
- ❏ It promotes accuracy in provision of cure and lessens the possibility of error.
- ❏ It helps the health personnel to make the best use of their time by avoiding overlapping activities.

The number and nature of reports will depend of what is required by the controlling body and the nursing councils. The preparations of such reports should be done very carefully and accurately as the date they give is frequently used for the purpose of planning and evaluation at state or national level. If the report is submitted on a structural form, the questions asked should be read carefully to avoid delay caused by returning them for clarification. It is important that such report are sent promptly as they may be required by the authority called for them to form a part of more comprehensive reports of the school in the state or country.

Type of Information for Annual Reports

- ❏ Factual data related to students, staff, clinical facilities physical facilities, administration and curriculum.
- ❏ Developments in the school program since the last report.
- ❏ Proposal and plans for future development.

All the schools and colleges have to report the records to the university.

Characteristics of Good Report

The characteristics of a good report are follows:

- ❏ **Promptness:** Reports should be made promptly to serve their purpose well such as condition of the patient or an accident report.
- ❏ **Organization:** All important points are mentioned in a logical manner. Before going to next patient or client, information about one should be complete.
- ❏ **Clarity:** Clearly stated what happened; how it was dealt, and what remains to be done.
- ❏ **Correction:** Giving correct information to prevent serious mistakes in providing continued efficient nurse care.
- ❏ **Brevity:** Report should be concise and complete, omit unnecessary words and statements should be concise and complete, omit unnecessary words and statements.
- ❏ **A good oral report:** It is always clearly expressed and presented with emphasis on all important points.
- ❏ **Objectivity:** Presentation of facts and not personal feeling include medication, treatment, and care given up to that time and what is to be given further. The constant exchange of information is essential to provide good patient care.

Types of Reports

Oral

Oral reports are given when information for immediate use and not for permanency and based on martial included in a written report.

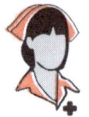

- Oral reports are sometimes used in an emergency and followed by written report.
- Oral report is made by the nurse who is assigned patient care to another nurse who is going to relieve her.
- A definite time and place needs to be arranged so that report can be given without interruption.
- The ward sister makes oral report to the matron and doctor. Sometimes nurses have to leave the ward to attend the meeting or classes and they have to handover the charge of patient to some other nurse. At that time, they should give complete report to the nurse relieving them. It must include medication, treatment, care given up to that time and what is to be given further. The constant exchange of information is essential to provide good patient care.

Written

While most reporting is done orally between the staff, certain reports need to be written. The important reports that are written in the ward are as follows:

- **Twenty four hours report (day, evening and night report):** The purpose of 24 hours report is to provide information about the patient to the head nurse, the ward nurses, night nurses, nursing office, day and night supervisors.
- **Census report:** Daily census or the number of patients in the hospital at midnight provides important source material for hospital statistics. Nurses should be very careful because single mistake in the census makes the entire census report incorrect.
- **Birth and death report:** Birth and death report are sent to the governmental authorities for registration within the specified period of time.
- **Anecdotal reports:** An anecdotal is a brief description of an incident. A written record regarding some observation about a person or about work without interpretation or criticism is called anecdotal. Anecdotes of both favorable and unfavorable incident have to be recorded. It helps the head nurse/clinical instructor to evaluate the program of the individual. Some important points to be kept in mind while writing anecdotal report are as follows:
  - The anecdote report should contain only what one has seen or heard by herself.
  - It should contain the date and time of observation, the name of the person who concerned.
  - Her ability to shoulder responsibility and work with others.
  - Ability to use safety measures to protect patients and workers.
  - Understanding and application of theoretical knowledge to practice.
  - Not even a smallest incident should be omitted from the report.
  - Before evaluation, a number of observations of similar behaviors are necessary. Then only, we can get the real picture of the person.

Reports of Mistakes and Accidents

Mistakes and accidents usually occur due to carelessness of individuals, but sometimes occur in spite of all precautions taken by the hospital administration to prevent them but report has to be made of each accident. It should be complete, clear and accurate because it is of legal value. Report should be filled in the nursing superintendent's office or hospital administration and investigated for prevention of such accident in future. The report should contain the name and age of the person, the exact time and place, a description how it occurred, precautions taken.

ASSESS YOURSELF

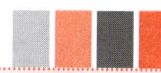

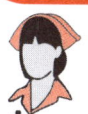

1. Describe hospital, types of hospital and the safety measures which should be taken care in the hospitals.

2. Explain leadership styles.

3. Write the meaning, types and importance of records and reports?

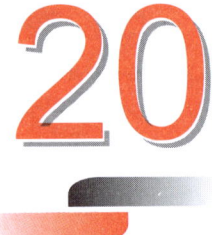

20
Management of Equipment and Supplies

Learning Objective

 Discuss the importance of maintaining supplies and equipment for effective administration.

Key Terms

⊷ **Inventory:** List of all articles.
⊷ **Procurement:** Security.
⊷ **Buffer stock:** Minimum stock to be kept.

Functional, accurate and safe clinical equipment is an essential requirement in the provision of health services. Well-maintained equipment will give nurse greater confidence in the reliability of its performance and contribute to a high standard of client care. Equipment management is an important issue for safety and cost in hospital management.

The term "equipment" means all items necessary for the functioning of all services of the hospital including accounting and records maintenance of buildings, laundry, nursing units, etc. both movable and fixed equipment are required for the hospital.

Supplies are those items that are used up or consumed, hence the term consumable is used for supplies. The supplies in hospital include drugs, surgical goods (disposables, glass wares) chemicals, antiseptics, food materials, stationeries, the linen supply, etc.

Nursing is a vital aspect of health care and needs to be properly organized. The director of nursing or his/her representative evaluates periodically the adequacy of facilities in terms of patients and personal needs. He or she requests after discussion with hospital administration, regarding any new facilities to be installed or if any expansion of facilities is required. Safe and effective care is evidenced by the development and use of inventories of equipment and standards for supplies. The availability of supplies in relation to storage and economical use of supplies. The director of nursing participates in joint planning session regarding expansion of facilities and services.

MAINTENANCE OF EQUIPMENT AND SUPPLIES

Proper maintenance of equipment is essential to obtain sustained benefits and to preserve capital investment. Equipment must be maintained in working order and calibrated for effectiveness and accuracy. Proper maintenance has a direct impact on quality of care.

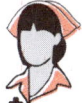

De Commissioning

- ❑ Repair existing old equipment
- ❑ Dismantle old units if required

Working of Departments Related to Equipment and Supply

- ❑ Purchase and store department.
- ❑ Equipment maintenance and repair department.

Each hospital has separate department/workshop for maintaining and repairing equipment. A biomedical engineer is usually appointed to supervise this important activity.

Careful handling, periodical cleaning, servicing disinfecting and repair helps to prolong life of equipment and other articles. The operation and service manuals supplied along with the equipment should be kept safe in purchasing department.

Duplicate copies may be supplied to the department. Each hospital should set up a condemnation committee to review the articles that are to be disposed off, when the articles cannot be used.

Management of Equipment and Supplies

No doubt the maintenance of equipment and supplies is one of the major work in the hospital set up but some of the following steps help and plays important role in managing the equipment and supplies.

Ordering Equipment and Supplies

The ordering helps us in setting the order of priorities. Based on the past experience and going through the catalogue, prepare a requisition from mentioning details and specifications place on order in the face of your requirements.

Storing Equipment

After getting equipment, it is the responsibility to store; prevent the equipment from theft, and breakage.

It is the job of the manager to see that storing should be done well and maintenance of proper accounting practices have been adopted through stock ledgers.

Issuing Equipment Supplies

When issuing an equipment to a particular department, after receiving the same, the concerned department bears responsibility of managing and controlling the properly. A material and stores manager is required to take care of the issue voucher since the person receiving or signing the voucher bears accountability. We have to keep the copy of the voucher.

Controlling and Maintaining Equipment and Supplies

After issuing the responsibility shift to the receiving person or the head of the department. He should make sure that equipment issued to the various departments are used in a right fashion, maintained properly and keeping up process is found regular. Should avoid misusing and unusing of equipment.

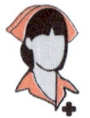

Coding and Standardization

We have to store a good number of items. The coding process would help in identifying particular equipment. Coding is done by classifying the items on functional basic. After coding, a catalog mentioning details of the codes should be maintained for references.

Usage and Maintenance

Every effort must be made at all levels to utilize the supplies in the most conscientious manner and avoid any form of wastage.

Proper maintenance and continuous availability should be make sure. Disposal of condemnation articles should be done.

❑ In the proper way through proper channel.
❑ **Pilferage:** Theft of material is not very uncommon.

Items may be pilfered by transporter, receiver, store personnel or the users.

Handing Over and Taking Over of Inventory

An inventory is a list of all the articles in the ward. It should include a clear description of each article and quantity that should be in the ward. It is always better to specify the articles by size, number and groups for listing the material like articles, linen, metal wire, and furnitures, etc. Some times the cost of the item is also mentioned. To organize the handing over and taking over of inventory is also known as inventory accounting system.

Mainly two types of systems are used to keep the account of the inventory. They are as follows:

1. Perpetual inventory system
2. Periodic inventory system

Perpetual Inventory System

Perpetual means continuous. Perpetual inventory system implies continuous maintenance of stock records and in its broad sense it covers both continuous stock taking as well as up to date recording of stores books.

Perpetual inventory system may be defined as a method of recording stores balances after every receipt and issue to facilitate regular checking and to obviate closing down for stock taking. This is a system where as organization keeps continuous moment-to-moment records of the number, value and type of inventories that it has.

Features

❑ This system updates inventory accounts after each purchase
❑ Inventory subsidiary ledger is updated after each transaction
❑ Inventory quantities are updated continuously.

Parts

This system comprise of three parts:

1. **Bin card:** Bin card is quantitative record of receipts, issues and closing balances of items of stores.

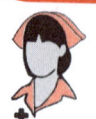

2. **Store ledgers:** Store ledgers are very useful inventory control system. It consists of leaf card for easy removal and insertion and useful in maintaining all costly items.
3. **Continues stock taking:** In this method limited items are verified. The items are selected based on their utility. Selected numbers of items are collected everyday and matched with the ledger book and bin card.

Periodic Inventory System

Periodic means at certain points in time. A periodic inventory system implies when the quantity on inventory on hand is determined on periodically such as once a month, quarterly or at the beginning and end of each year and does not have an accurate record of the inventories in between these points. This system does not keep continuous moment-to-moment records of inventories.

Features

❑ All acquisitions of inventory during the accounting period are recorded by debits to purchases account.
❑ The total in the purchases account at the end of the accounting period added to the cost of the inventory on hand at the beginning of the period.
❑ Inventory subsidiary ledger is not updated after each purchase of inventory.
❑ Inventory quantities are not updated continuously rather updated on periodic basis.

Table 1: A sample form for ward inventory

S. No.	Item name	Specifications	Number	Cost (in ₹)	Date of purchase	Condition at the time of receiving
1	Bed locker	Steel	8	800/- per locker	12–2–16	New
2						
3						

Indent and Ordering for Supplies and Equipment

Indent or requisition is a written order for supplies and equipment. A wise ordering is necessary to keep sufficient amount of supplies and equipment at hand. A requisition may be written by the ward incharge or person responsible for handling supply and equipment. Before ordering he must check the number at hand and then, consider the expected needs and write the requisition.

Supply System

Some hospitals have central supply system and separate department where equipment and supplies are stored and dispensed to the wards on loan on exchange basis. The type of material that is kept in center supply varies from hospital to hospital. In some hospitals, the center supply deals only with sterile supplies and articles which are not used frequently and are kept in central supply. Commonly and frequently used articles may be stored in ward. In some hospitals all types of equipment such as oxygen suction, traction, I/V sets, procedure tray, catheters, etc. are stored in central supply. At the time of treatment required supply can be obtained by sending requisition.

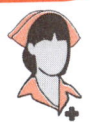

Factors in Determining Amount and Type of Material Supplied from Central Supply Department

- Cost of equipment and frequency of use in a particular unit. Few sets are needed where use is limited.
- The ease and rapidity with which equipment can be obtained.
- The facilities in the ward for care, sterilization and storage of equipment. This includes the personnel to clean and test the articles.
- The facilities in the central supply for the same function.
- The amount of up keep involved and technical ability needed to achieve it.

Advantages of Central Supply System

Every hospital these days has some type of central supply services because:

- The greatest advantage of this system is to increase the efficiency and conserving the time of nurses.
- Smaller number and less frequently used articles are necessary, if they are issued from central supply department.
- Mechanical defects are detected early and articles can be repaired before the damage is great.
- The facilities for cleaning in central supply are better than possible in the ward.
- Big advantage is that set and trays prepared centrally are uniform and comply with established standards.
- Work of cleaning and wrapping can be done by non-nursing personnel, thus saving the nurses time for nursing activities.
- Sterilization of equipment can be controlled by a few persons in a central department.
- Lessen the responsibility of ward incharge due to centralization of stock.

Disadvantages of Central Supply System

The only disadvantage of central supply services is the possible delay in obtaining material. If everything is centralized, however, this can be overcome by having each ward stock and supplies and sets sufficient in number to meet daily requirements. In the same way, the equipment which might be needed in an emergency for a particular service can be stocked in minimum amount in the ward.

PROBLEM SOLVING: PROCESS AND APPROACH

Steps and Methods of Dealing with Supplies and Equipment

The problem solving process deals with supplies of equipment has the following steps:

- Budgeting and material planning/demand estimation
- Procurement/Purchasing
- Receipt and inspection
- Inventory control
- Maintenance and repair
- Disposal and condemnation

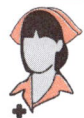

It is like a cyclic process and the steps get one after the other (Fig. 1).

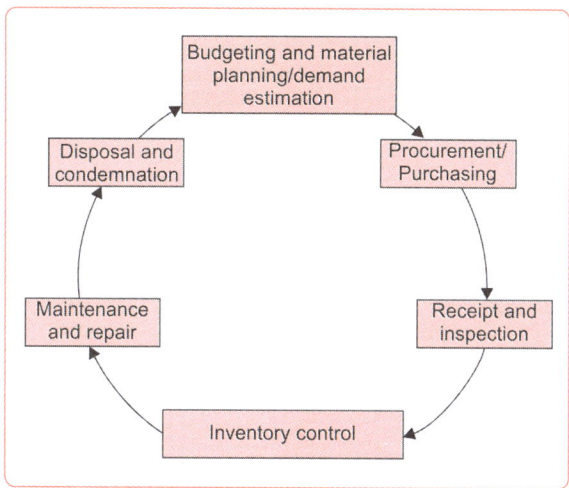

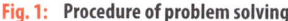

Fig. 1:   Procedure of problem solving

Budgeting and Material Planning

Based on the data of past levels of performance and on anticipated activity/plans, capital equipment, consumables and supplies to be procured during the year ahead can be projected department wise. This is the budget which should be prepared annually. At periodic intervals carry out a budgetary appraisal and determine the variance between actual and the budget.

Materials in the hospital may be requisitioned:

❑   For an urgent/immediate use or in anticipation of need.

❑   On a one time basis or repeatedly and continuously to replenish the stock.

❑   As a single unit or as a bulk requirement.

Procurement

After determining supply requirement the next step in material management is security or procuring the needed articles. State governments have laid down detailed rules and regulations regarding procurements of materials. Many states have medical stores which are centralized agencies for procurement of drugs and supplies.

The main objectives of procurement are like, it helps in having continuous supply of materials, maintaining standards of quality, avoidance of duplication and waste, etc. It helps in maintenance of interpersonal, interdepartmental, and vender relations. The maintenance of proper records is must in procurement.

Procurement can be done by centralized and decentralized purchasing. Following principles can be kept in mind while purchasing:

■   Tight quality
■   Right quantity
■   Right time
■   Right source
■   Right price

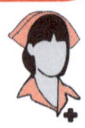

Receipt and Inspection

It is done when the stores orders are received in the store. Material inspection is necessary to ensure quality of material received. Whenever an item is delivered the same is verified in the presence of the store incharge, representative of the supplier and representative from the purchase committee of the hospital. Verification is done to ensure that the item is as per the order placed. If verifications are not satisfactory then actions are taken as per the terms of MOU.

Inventory Control

Inventory control deals with storage and distribution issues. After the verification of the purchased items the items came to the store for storage, issue and distribution. Proper storage ensures that fills the time of issue for usage, the supplies are adequately preserved to prevent loss or damage when material is in the store. These materials should be taken care and looked after properly.

Inventory control is must for minimizing and control of investment on materials. There are many concepts for the inventory control which are as follows:

❏ **Cyclic system:** This is the simplest way of inventory in which at the periodic time the order is placed according to the material in store and rate of consumption.

❏ **Two-bin system:** There are two bins of inventory stock. One large bin is there to have sufficient stock to meet demands during intervals between arrival of order quantity and placing of next order, i.e. when the first bin is empty then the material is shifted from second bin to first bin and new arrived material is stocked.

❏ **Lead time:** This is the time period between the order placed and the material received. The amount which is consumed between this time should be stocked in the inventory. The longer lead time the higher is inventory level.

❏ **Buffer stocks/minimum stock of safety:** As the name indicates it is the minimum amount of material which is to be kept for the time of the inventory ordered and the inventory received. This amount of stock should be kept to avoid a stock out in case of more demand.

❏ **Record point level or ROP:** In record point level the order is placed when the stock comes to a level from where it is predetermined the time of arrival of the material.

❏ **Minimum stock:** It is the stock at minimum level and beyond that emergency can occur at any time.

❏ **Economic order quantity:** This is the quantity in which the cost of carrying the material is same as the cost of ordering.

❏ **ABC analysis:** It is found that in most of inventories some items have a much higher annual usage value than others. ABC analysis separates inventories into ABC items. In order to make such an analysis the list of all the stored items and their annual consumption in value is tabulated on the basis of the latest available records. Each individual item and its annual consumption values are listed separately and then this list is rearranged in the descending order.

Approximately account for 70–80% of the value are placed under category A, 20–25% in category B and 5–10% value in category C.

Items of "A" should be strictly supervised, whereas least control may be exercised such as "C" category, items of "B" category require only moderate control. Such control is known as ABC analysis.

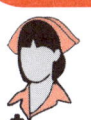

- ❑ **VED analysis:** Items may be classified as vital, essential and desirable. It is used for medical stores, spare parts, inventory, etc.

  Essential items are those, the absence of which cannot be tolerated more than one day or so.
  - ■ The desirable items are those which are definitely needed but with their absence, the work can continue.
  - ■ Vital drugs should be stocked adequately to meet emergencies. Desirable drugs have substitute and are easily available in the market.

- ❑ **FSN analysis:** Stock can be classified into the fast moving items or the more consumable items and less consumable items or slow moving items. The slow or non-moving items should be taken care proper for their expiry or damage.

- ❑ **Turnover of inventory:** It is quantitative measurement means how much of the total inventory is issued or replaced. The rate is calculated as:

$$\text{Turnover inventory rate} = \frac{\text{Total rupee value of supplies}}{\text{Rupee value of closing stock}}$$

- ❑ **Physical inventory:** This is the way of verification of the stock. Each thing in the inventory is physically checked and matched with the records. This may be in term of objects, drugs or it may be in terms of rupees. This is done once and twice in a year. During this time issue of the articles is avoided so it should take as less time as possible.

Issue and Distribution

Hospital or any organization cannot run smoothly without the uninterrupted supply of the material and the stores have this main role. This supply etc. can only be done with a systematic procedure and a proper recording of the material received and issued. The stores have the responsibility of smooth issue of accurate stock, status report, and timely detection of discrepancies and prompt clearance of goods inward notes to expedite bill payments etc.

Distribution usually involves transportation to various unit or health care delivery system. It is an intricate process focusing on distribution of the right at right time and at right place. Usually two methods are adopted:

1. Requisition system
2. Par level system.

The requisition system is the most widely used method in Indian hospitals. Each user department maintain and keeps track of its inventories. Periodically or when requisition is prepared and sent to stores which deliver the requisitioned items.

Medical equipment, computer systems, etc. are purchased and directly installed at the site of operation. In that case after successful installation of the item, the transaction is recorded in the material issue register.

Maintenance and Repair

Maintenance and repair will go side by side of various equipment. Proper maintenance helps reduce the losses and breakdown of the equipment. It is important to know that 'A stich in time saves the nine'.

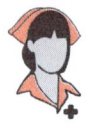

Disposal and Condemnation

Surplus products and nonfunctional equipment which are functional but absolute or nonfunctional and absolute or beyond economic repair, functional but hazardous, functional but no longer required will require disposal. It is important to decrease in holding costs and in storage capacity. All the hospitals have condemnation committee. Disposal is done by sold to other hospitals, to scrape dealers.

The hospital also undertakes periodic write off of the items which are not fit to be used. The store maintains complete details about each item in the hospital including their expiry dates. The store immediately disposes any expired items.

The user department informs the store in writing about any equipment etc. which are to be disposed. The store immediately makes assignment for removal of the same from the user department. Before removing the equipment cannibalization of parts is done so that the usable parts of discarded machine can be used in future for other machine of same type.

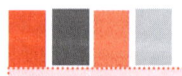 **ASSESS YOURSELF**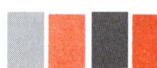

1. Define inventory. As a head nurse, how will you maintain equipment and supplies of your ward.

2. What is center supply system? What are the advantages and disadvantages of this system?

3. Describe problem solving process and approaches.

Cost of Health Care

21

Learning Objectives

- To discuss the cost, type of cost, health finance.
- To describe the national health plans.
- To discuss about insurance schemes.

Key Terms

- **Cost of health care:** Health financial systems.
- **MNP:** Minimum need program.
- **Health insurance:** Insurance against health.
- **ESI:** Employees State Insurance.

Good health is the fundamental right to every human being. The mission of good health is social justice which entitle people to basic necessities such as adequate income and health protection. The health status of community is associated with several factors such as health care access economic conditions, social and environmental issues and culture practice. Economics affects all aspects of health.

Although efforts have been made to control the cost of health care, these costs continue to increase employees legislations, insurances and health care provide to collaborate in efforts to resolve the issues surrounding to deliver best health care costs.

From the above discussion we have to see what is health care and what is cost? Let us see what is cost first?

Cost is defined as a set of procedures for determining the cost of the product or service and various activities involved in the manufacture and sales, for planning and measuring performance. Therefore the functions of cost are:

- To determine and analyze the cost, which helps in evaluating the operating efficiency at each stage.
- Accumulation and utilization of cost data.
- Aid to management, to arrive at the cost of production, work order processes, etc.

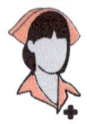

TYPES OF COST

Opportunity Cost

Opportunity cost is that cost which a person gets in any field of work.

Fixed Cost

Fixed cost is the sum total of expenditure incurred by the producer on the purchase of hiring of fixed factors of production. It may be defined as the sum total of all the fixed costs incurred for the activity to be carried out, or the program fixed cost do not change with the change in the quality of output, volume of output even if the output is zero or the output is maximum fixed cost remains the same.

Variable Cost

Variable costs are the sum total of all the variable costs incurred in the program or the activity. These costs are incurred on the use of variable factors. It varies with the variation of the output of the production. When output changes these cost also changes.

Average Cost

Average cost is the cost per unit of output produced. It is also called cost of production. It is total cost divided by the output. Average cost is equal to the average fixed cost plus average variable cost.

Marginal Cost

Marginal cost is the change in total cost by producing one more or one less unit of output.

Actual Cost

Actual cost can be expressed in terms of discomforts, sacrifice and efforts undergone in the production of goods.

COST BENEFIT

It is a method of comparing the cost of providing a service with the gain accruing or likely to accrue from it. In other words, it pertains to the ratio of the benefit to the cost. It is often not possible to measure benefits of a particular program accurately in terms of monetary gains, disease prevented or outcome death prevented, birth avoided, etc. Thus, it is a technique of measuring various alternatives. In practice, it is mainly used to justify a particular health service/program.

What we are pointing out that, 'one time' may be composed with benefits a spread overtime. The main problem in cost-benefit analysis is that the cost and benefits are likely to be spread overtime and are usually not measured at the same time. As the time passes the value of benefit thus decrease in the monitory value. To overcome this problem the economist uses the value of discounted rate for convince. The scope for this method in health management is limited.

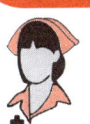

Cost Benefits Analysis

Cost benefit analysis is a tool with great potential for the decision maker so long as he or she recognizes the difficulty in determining the true costs and benefits of various alternatives. This tool can be especially useful when trying to decide between alternative expenditure of money.

A cost benefit ratio (Z) is defined as the ratio of the value of benefits of an alternative to the value of alternative cost.

$$Z = \frac{\text{Present value of economic benefits}}{\text{Present value of economic cost}}$$

Cost benefit analysis is designed to consider the social costs and benefits attributable to the project. The benefits are expressed in monetary terms to determine whether a given program is economically sound, and to select the best out of several programs.

COST EFFECTIVENESS

Cost effective methods are those that search for least costly way of achieving a defined result. Cost effective analyzes are easier to make, as that is clear. It helps the administrator in managing his health resources at the local level. The problem is to find the way of achieving the objective at lower cost.

Cost of Health Care

From the above discussion, now we know what cost is? It is the time to see the cost of health care now. Efforts have been implemented some cost containment strategies including health promotion and illness prevention activities, managed care system and alternative insurance delivery systems.

Economics deals with efficient allocation of resources. It determines which alternatives represent the most efficient use of resources. But social, ethical and moral questions must be considered to determine whether the most efficient allocation is socially acceptable. Economic resources are sources of support that are in short supply, such as money, material and employees. The objective for budgeting is to ensure attainment of desired goals by using the fewest possible resources. Resources are sometimes called assets and may be tangible or intangible. Money is tangible asset, whereas agency reputation and employee morale are intangible assets.

Budgeting is the allocation of scarce resources on the basis of forecasted needs for proposed activities over specified time period. The budget document is a numerical expression of an agency's expected income and planned expenditure for a specified period of time.

A unit of service is a specific measure of health care work that a department delivers to customers or clients. The following units of services have been used to measure medical productivity: patients per day, home visits, clinic visits, surgical procedures. A program is a series of activities that function together to facilitate obtaining some desired goal. Four types of expenditures may be defined for a program that are:

1. **Past expenditure:** Funds that were expended for the program during a previous budget cycle.
2. **Permitted expenditure:** Funds that have been authorized for application to the program by the agency's chief executive or governing body.
3. **Proposed expenditure:** Funds that have been requested by an operating manager to support program during a future budget period.

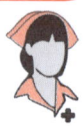

4. **Predicted expenditure:** Costs/funds for the program that have been forecasted for 1 to 5 years by the manager responsible for its administration.

HEALTH FINANCE

Finance is that branch of economics which is concerned with the study of revenue and expenditure of public authorities. It focuses on how government policies of taxation and public expenditure affect the economy and the welfare of the people living in the country. In other words finance studies, how public authorities raise revenue and incur expenditure so that the society may get maximum social benefit. Besides the revenue and expenditure activities of the public authorities, finance also studies how and when government raises public department manages financial administration of the government and maintains stability and growth of the economy and manages distribution of resources between different layers of the government.

Hence some definitions of the finance can be studies as follows:

❑ Finance deals with the income and expenditure of public authorities and with the manner in which the one is adjusted with the other.

❑ Finance means the financial resources or income and expenditure of the government of a country.

❑ Finance studies the economic activities of government as a unit

❑ It is one of the subjects that lie between economics and politics.

Up to now we are clear that what the finance means. Now we will consider about the health financing.

Health Financing System in India

People consider using the government health services as the last resort, after depleting all their financial resources in the private sector. Besides scarcity of funds, the government health system in India suffers from the problem of displaced priority. The political and bureaucratic leadership and specialist lobbies try to keep pumping funds to the large urban hospitals so that the state of art medical care is available to their elite population.

Many families are ruined in the process of financing for the medical treatment for their near and dear ones. The medical insurances in India are very short and out of the reach of common people.

There are health facilities of different government departments as army medical corps, railways medical corps, hospital of public sector units and ESI.

These facilities normally cater to the health needs of specific clients. However, in the situation of disaster these facilities can be used by and are a great support to the common people. The primary source of the funds/money is public. On the basis of control over funds, health finances are derived from four avenues.

1. **Government funds:** Government has the responsibility to facilitate healthy and prosperous life of people for whom it works. For meeting this basic objective, governments have to carry out a wide range of functions such as security, infrastructure, enactment and enforcement of laws, education, health and nutrition. Each of these sectors often competes with each other for resources. Government does recognize the fact that health is the precondition for prosperity and development. They invest in their health systems with great priority.

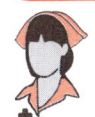

In almost all developed countries, governments spend heavily on health, even though the majority of their citizens are in a position to pay for health services. A few underdeveloped countries, who have also considered health a priority issue, have achieved accelerated development rates. In rest of the countries, the government expenditure on health does not meet the needs of the system, yet the government funds remain the largest organized resource pool for health systems. These funds are directly paid by the patient's family for receiving services or buying medicines.

2. **Private out of pocket funds:** This is the crudest form of the private health system includes large corporation hospitals, nursing homes and individual practitioners. However, the concentration of private medical facilities is centered grossly around urban areas. The poor and rural population has to rely on a large number of unqualified practitioner and traditional practitioners. The health services in the private hospitals are very expensive and have to borne out of pocket financing of health system. In this system poor are deprived of quality care and have to compromise with the other imported needs of the family like nutrition, education, house, etc. The out of pocket funds are the choice for only those who have a good paying capacity. This type of the financing is very prevalent in India and other developing countries where the government systems are not up to mark or sick. What so ever it is this type of the health financing should be discouraged.

3. **Insurance:** In 1965, the federal government enacted the first movement towards universal health care coverage. As the popularity and benefits of employer—provided insurance plans were recognized. It became evident that health care of some segments of society was being neglected. Insurance has been identified as one of the most successful means of health financing, especially for medical care. Health insurance could be operated either by public or by private operators. Government operated insurance usually aim at providing low cost coverage to large population whereas the private operators work for high profit margins and are thus more interested in high income groups.

    Government operated insurance usually aims at providing low cost coverage to a large population whereas the private operators work for high profit margins and are thus more interested in high income groups. Government operated insurance is generally part of the social security network and is mandatory for target population.

4. **Donations:** Although donations play a very important role in the health systems especially in emergencies and deprived areas. This fact has yet to receive the research attention it deserves. The reasons could be nonavailability of adequate data and unpredictability of these funds.

NATIONAL HEALTH PLANS

National health planning is the planning in which India has been the pioneer not only at the time of independence but even earlier. Since "health" is an important contributory factor in the utilization of manpower, the Planning Commission gave considerable importance to health program in the five-year plans for purpose of planning, the health sector has been divided in the following sub-sectors:

❑ Water supply and sanitation
❑ Control of communicable diseases
❑ Medical education, training and research
❑ Medical care included hospitals, dispensaries and primary health centers
❑ Public health services

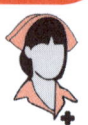

❑ Family planning
❑ Indigenous system of medicine

The main objectives of the health program during the five-year plans are as follows:

❑ Control or eradication of major communicable diseases
❑ Strengthening of the basic health services through the establishment of primary health care centers and subcenters
❑ Population control
❑ Development of health manpower resources.

To all above basic objectives and the subsectors have received due consideration in five-year plans. However, the emphasis has been changed from plan to plan depending upon the felt-needs of the people and technical considerations. To give effect to a better coordination between the center and state governments, a bureau of planning was constituted in 1965 in ministry of health, Government of India. The main function of this bureau is completion of National health five-year plans.

The health plan is implemented at various levels.

■ Center level
■ State level
■ District level
■ Block level
■ Village level

FIVE-YEAR PLANS

The five-year plans were conceived to rebuilt rural India.

First Five-Year Plan (1951–56)

Prior to the starting of first five-year plan the health status of the Indian people was very low, economy was low, had inadequate financial resources and lack of training to the health personal.

While considering these draw backs and facts a seven-point public health program with the following priorities formed the basis of first five-year plan from 1951 to 1956.

❑ Provision of water supply and sanitation
❑ Control of malaria
❑ Preventive health care of the rural population through health units and mobile units
❑ Health services for mother and children
❑ Education, training and health education
❑ Self-sufficiency in drugs and equipment
❑ Family planning and population control.

During this plan period the public-sector outlay was ₹2,356 crore of which 140 crore were allotted for health programs. The actual expenditure, however, amounted to ₹1960 and ₹101 crore respectively.

Second Five-Year Plan (1956–61)

The second five-year plan was continuation of the development efforts commenced in the first plan. It included all communicable diseases in addition to control of malaria.

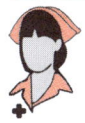

The specific objectives were:

❑ Establishment of institutional facilities to serve as a basis from which services could be rendered to the people both locally and in surrounding territories.
❑ Development of technical manpower through appropriate training programs.
❑ Intensifying measures to control widely spread communicable diseases.
❑ Encouraging active campaign for environmental hygiene.
❑ Provision of family planning and other supporting services for raising health standard of the people.

The different areas emphasized during the second five-year plan were:

❑ Health care services in rural and urban areas
❑ Medical education and training
❑ Medical research
❑ Indigenous system of medicine
❑ Control of communicable diseases
❑ MCH and family planning
❑ Health education

During this period, the public sector outlay was ₹4800 crore of which ₹225 crore were allotted to the health programs. The actual expenditure was ₹4672 crore and ₹215 crore respectively.

Third Five-Year Plan (1961–1966)

The objectives of the third five-year plan were in time with the first and second five-year plans except that integration of public health with material and child welfare, nutrition and health education was planned. In general, the third five-year plan focused on the following areas:

❑ Water supply and environmental sanitation
❑ Health care (hospitals and dispensaries)
❑ Control of communicable diseases
❑ Medical education, research and training
❑ Other services—health education, school health, MCH, mental health and health insurance
❑ ISM and family planning.

During this period public sector outlay was ₹7500 crore of which ₹341.80 crore allotted for health programs. The actual expenditure, however, amounted to ₹8577 crore and ₹357 crore respectively.

Annual Plans (1966–69)

The fourth annual plan which should have been started from 1966 had been postponed till 1969 due to some economic and unavoidable situations like Indo-Pak war. During this intervening period (1966–69) war covered by annual plans with an outlay of ₹6756 crore in public sector of which the expenditure on health program was ₹316 crore.

Fourth Five-Year Plan (1969–74)

In this five-year plan certain objectives of the Mudaliar Committee were the base, in relation to health. These were as follows:

❑ To provide an effective base for health services in rural areas by strengthing the primary health centers.

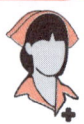

- ❑ Strengthing of subdivisional and district hospitals to provide effective referral services for primary health center.
- ❑ Expansion of the medical and nursing education and training of paramedical personnel to meet the minimum technical manpower requirements.

    In the fourth five-year plan, public health and medical program had been divided into the following broad categories.
    - ▪ Medical education, training and research
    - ▪ Control of communicable diseases
    - ▪ Medical care included hospitals, dispensaries and PHCs
    - ▪ Other public health services
    - ▪ Indigenous system of medicine.

During this period the revised estimation of public sector outlay was ₹16,774 crore out of which 7.2%, i.e. ₹1156 crore was allotted to the health sector.

Fifth Five-Year Plan (1974–79)

The primary objective of this fifth five-year plan was "to provide minimum public health facilities integrated with family planning and nutrition for vulnerable groups especially children, pregnant woman and feeding mothers."

The emphasis of the plan was on removing imbalance in respect of medical facilities and strengthening the health infrastructure in rural areas, specific objectives to be presumed during the plan were:

- ❑ Increasing accessibility of health services to rural areas
- ❑ Correcting regional imbalance
- ❑ Further development of referral services by removing deficiencies, in district and subdivisional hospitals
- ❑ Integration of health, family planning and nutrition
- ❑ Intensification of the control and eradication of communicable diseases especially malaria and smallpox.
- ❑ Quantitative improvement in the education and training of health personnel by converting unipurpose workers to multipurpose workers.
- ❑ Development of referral services by providing specialists attention to common diseases in rural areas.

    This fifth five-year plan was launched on 1st, April 1, 1974 with an outlay of ₹37,250 crore in the public sector out of which ₹3277 crore were allotted to health sector.

Minimum Need Program (MNP)

Minimum need program (MNP) was first introduced in fifth five-year plan to combat poverty. The state has a duty to provide a basic need of life to every citizen in terms of health, food, education, water, shelter, etc. MNP is the expression of the commitment of the government for the socio-economic development of the community, particularly the underserved and under privileged segment of population. Government considers investment in health as an investment in human resources development and as such primary health care forms an essential and integral component of the MNP. It is a broad intersectoral, master plan for providing the minimum basic needs of people of land and includes the following aspects in revised MNP of 1978.

- ❑ Elementary education
- ❑ Adult education

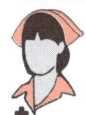

- Rural health
- Rural water supply
- Rural roads
- Rural electrification
- House site→house for rural landless
- Environment improvement of slums
- Nutrition

The basic principles to be observed in implementation of minimum need program are:

- The facilities in MNP are provided on priority basis. First only in those areas which are under served so that the disparity from area to area is eliminated and every segment of population is assured of minimum essential facility.
- All the facilities under MNP are provided as package to a broad intersectoral area. This would insure a later impact of the facility provided.

Health Sector Minimum Need Program

Health in its wider concept cannot be attained by health sector alone. Economic development, antipoverty measures, food production and distribution, drinking water supply, sanitation, housing, environmental protection and education contribute to health and have the common goal of human development.

Health services are an integral part of overall social and economic development and necessarily rest on proper co-ordination at all level between the health's of all other sector.

Centrally sponsored (100%) scheme

- Health guide scheme
- Establishment of subcenters
- Basic training of multipurpose worker
- Training of specialists, technical and other paramedical staff required for rural medical services
- Training of community health officers

Centrally assisted scheme (50–50 basis)

- Multipurpose workers scheme

State scot scheme

- Subsidiary health centers
- Primary health centers
- Community health centers or upgraded PHCs

Sixth Five-Year Plan (1980–85)

The main objectives of the sixth five-year plan were as follows:

- Progressive reduction in the incidence of poverty and unemployment
- To step up the rate of growth of the Indian economy
- Promoting policies for controlling the population growth through voluntary acceptance of the small family norm.

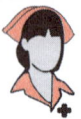

❑ To improve the quality of life of the people in general through "minimum need program". The sixth plan laid emphasis on health care, control of communicable diseases, hospital and dispensaries in urban/rural areas, medical education, research, training ISM and homeopathy, other programs and family welfare.

❑ The total investment on this plan was ₹97,500 crore for the total as health, family welfare and water supply and sanitation.

Seventh Five-Year Plan (1985–90)

The objectives of the seventh five-year plan have been formulated as part of the long-term strategy which seeks by the year 2000 to virtually eliminate poverty and illiteracy, achieve near full employment, secure satisfaction of the basic needs of food, clothing shelter and provide health for all.

Against the above background the current objective of the state and national health plan is to continue the reorganization of the health services infrastructure, already begun in the state five-year plan (1980–85) and strive towards the goal of health for all by the year 2000 through provision of universal primary health care to all sections of the society.

By the end of seventh five-year plan, it is envisaged that the infrastructure of primary health care as required on present population norms would be fully operational with regard to village health guides, primary health centers and subcenters used multipurpose health workers. Programs for the control of communicable diseases, of health services research and of health education will be strengthened. The universal immunization to be completed by the 1990. The family welfare program will be implemented with greater vigous so as to achieve couple protection, rate 42% by the end of seventh plan period with increased emphasis on female education and MCH services.

In keeping with the objectives of the international drinking water supply and sanitation decades (1988–91), the seventh plan aims to provide adequate drinking water facilities for the entire population both in urban and in rural area and sanitation facilities for 80% of the urban population and 25% of the rural population.

The public-sector outlay of ₹180,000 crore represent a massive public investment out of this national cake nearly ₹3392 crore are earmarked for health, ₹3922 crore for water supply and sanitation and ₹3256 crore for family welfare program. The targets to be achieved are laid down in national health policy.

Eighth Five-Year Plan (1992–97)

The ultimate goal of the eight five-year plan is the human development in many facets. It is towards fulfilling this goal that the eighth plan accords priority to the generation of adequate employment opportunities to achieve near full employment by the turn of the century building up of the people institutions, control of population growth, universalization of elementary education, eradication of illiteracy, provision of safe drinking water and primary health facilities to all, growth and diversification of agriculture to achieve self-sufficiency in food grains and generate surpluses for exports. So, in this five-year plan, employment generation, population control, literacy, education, health, drinking water and provision of adequate food and basic infrastructure are listed as priorities. All these aspects contribute to the health of the people.

In relation to health, this plan period has the following:

■ The "health for all" must take into account not only the high risk vulnerable groups but also focus sharply on underprivileged segments.

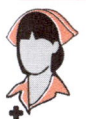

- Delivery of health services must undergo reorientation by emphasis the community-based system, these systems must be reflected in planning of infrastructure with about 30,000 population as a unit.

Hence, the aim of eighth five-year plan was "health for all paradigms" to towards "health for the underprivileged." Thus, plan priority emphasis is the need for a major thrust in improving qualitative aspects of personnel, such as motivation skills and managerial abilities of personnel, community participation and intersectoral coordination for health.

The total outlay money for eighth five-year plan was ₹798,000 crore from which ₹7575.92 crore for health, ₹6500 crore for family welfare and ₹16,711.03 crore for water supply and sanitation was used.

Ninth Five-Year Plan (1997–2002)

The ninth five-year plan is unique in a way that although the plan commenced from April 1, 1977, the formal ninth plan document finally received all the necessary clearance and was adopted only on February 19, 1998.

Today, India has a vast network of government, voluntary and private health infrastructure planned by large number of medical and paramedical persons. During the ninth plan, efforts will further intensify to improve the health status of population by optimizing coverage and quality of care by identifying the critical gaps in infrastructure, manpower, equipment, essential diagnostic reagents and drugs.

The approach during the ninth plan will be improved and enhance the quality of primary health care in urban and rural areas by providing an optimally functioning primary health care system as a part of basic minimum services and to improve the existing health care infrastructure. Primary, secondary and tertiary care setting through appropriate institutional strengthening and improvement of referral linkages.

The new initiatives in ninth plan are as follows:

- Horizontal integration of vertical programs.
- Develop disease surveillance and response mechanisms with focus on rapid recognition report and response at district level.
- Develop and implement integrated noncommunicable disease control program.
- Health assessment as part of environment impact assessment in development projects.
- Implement appropriate management system for emergency disaster and accidents.
- Screening for common nutritional deficiencies specially in vulnerable groups and initiate appropriate remedial measures.
- Reduction in population growth rate has been recognized as one of the priority objectives.
- Implementation of RCH program by effective MCH, increased access to contraceptive care, safe management of unwanted pregnancies, nutritional services to vulnerable groups, prevention and treatment of STD/UTI/RTI, reproductive health services for adolescence, treatment and prevention of gynecological problems, screening and treatment of cancers especially of uterine, cervix and breast.

₹859,200 crore was the total plan investment from which ₹10,818.40 crore for health and ₹15,120.20 crore for family welfare was utilized.

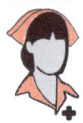

Tenth Five-Year Plan (2002–2007)

In the tenth five-year plan it was planned that the efforts will be further intensified to improve the health status of the population by optimizing coverage and quality of care. It will be done by identifying and rectifying the critical gaps in infrastructure, manpower, equipment, essential diagnostic reagents and drugs.

The services which should be rendered for minimum need program should be made better and easily available. Improvement of primary, secondary, tertiary services and referral services to be done.

The mentionable targets for tenth five-year plan and beyond are as follows:

- Reduction of poverty ratio by 5% point by 2007 and by 15% points by 2012.
- All children in school by 2003 and all children to complete five-years of schooling by 2007.
- Reduction in gender gaps in literacy and wage rates by at least 50% by 2007.
- Reduction in the decadal rate of population growth between 2001 and 2011 to 16.2%.
- Increase in literacy rate to 75% within the plan period.
- Reduction of maternal mortality ratio to 2/1000 live birth by 2007 and to 1 by 2012.
- Reduction of infant mortality rate to 45/100 live births by 2007 and to 28 by 2012.
- All villagers to have sustained access to potable drinking water within plan period.

The total outlay money ₹148,4131.30 crore and ₹31,020.30 crore for health and ₹27,12500 for family welfare is used.

Eleventh Five-Year Plan (2007–2012)

Eleventh five-year plane was started in 2007 to 2012. The eleventh five-year plan target was as follows:

- Accelerate growth rate of GDP from 8% to 10% and then maintain to 10% in the 12th plan in order to double per capita income by 2016–17.
- Increase agricultural GDP growth rate to 4% per year.
- Reduce educated unemployment to below 5%.
- Raise real wage rate of unskilled workers by 20%.

Objectives of Eleventh Five-Year Plan (2007–2012)

- To increase GDP growth to 10%
  - Increase agricultural GDP growth to 4% per year to ensure a wider spread of benefits.
  - Create 70 million new work opportunities.
  - Augment minimum standards of education in primary school.
  - Reduce infant mortality rate to 2 and malnutrition among children of age group 0–3 to half of its present level.
  - Ensure electricity connection to all villages and increase forest and tree cover by five per percentage points.

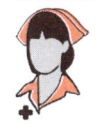

Twelfth Five-Year Plan (2012–2017)

Twelfth five-year plan is working in this time. The main objectives of the twelfth five-year plan are:

❑ Better performance in agriculture (at least 4% growth)
❑ Faster creation of job in manufacturing specification on a target for extra jobs to be created in this sector in next 5 years.
❑ Wider industrial growth to enhance employment.
❑ The creation of appropriate infrastructural facilities to enhance agricultural and manufacturing growth along with rural connectivity.
❑ Stronger efforts at health, education and skill development.
❑ Reforming the implementation of flagship programs to increase their effectiveness in achieving the objective of greater inclusion.
❑ Special challenges focused on vulnerable groups and backward regions. The need for a special focus on backward regions has been particularly urgent.

HEALTH INSURANCE

Health insurance is the insurance against the risk of incurring medical expanses among individuals. According to health insurance association of America, health insurance is defined as "coverage that provides for the payments of benefits as a result of sickness or injury. It includes insurance for excess from accident, medical expenses, disability, accidental death and disbursement".

A health insurance policy is:

❑ A renewable contract between the insurance provider (may be governmental or private) and individual in written form with selective terms and conditions.
❑ Individual and insurance provider both are satisfied with the terms and conditions.

Types of Health Insurance Policies

Health insurance in India typically pays for only inpatient hospitalization and for treatment in hospitals in India. Outpatient services are not under health policies in India. The first health policy in India was mediclaim policy. In 2000 government of India liberalized insurance and allowed private players into the insurance sector.

Broadly, the health insurance plans in India nowadays can be classified into three.
1. Hospitalization plans.
2. Hospital daily cash benefit plans.
3. Critical illness plans.

Under the Income Tax Act under section 80D, the insured person who takes out the policy can claim for tax deductions.

Some insurance schemes and their details are listed on next page which can give the detailed knowledge about the health insurances Table 1.

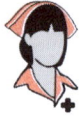

Table 1: Insurance schemes and their details

Scheme	Ministry	Date of launch	Outlay/ Status	Sector	Provisions
Aam Aadmi Bima Yojana	MoF	2007		Insurance	Scheme extends the benefit of life insurance coverage as well as coverage of partial and permanent disability to the head of the family or an earning member of the family of rural landless households and educational assistance to their children studying from 9th to 12th standard as an extended benefit
Atal Pension Yojana	MoF	May 9, 2015		Pension	Social sector scheme pertaining to pension sector
Bachat Lamp Yojna	MoP	2009		Electrification	Reduce the cost of compact fluorescent lamps
Central Government Health Scheme	MoHFW	1954		Health	Comprehensive medical care facilities to Central Government employees and their family members
Deendayal Disabled Rehabilitation Scheme	MoSJE	2003		[Social Justice]	Create an enabling environment to ensure equal opportunities, equity, social justice and empowerment of persons with disabilities
Deen Dayal Upadhyaya Gram Jyoti Yojana	MoP	2015		Rural Power Supply	It is a Government of India program aimed at providing 24 × 7 uninterrupted power supply to all homes in rural India
Digital India Program	MoC&IT	July 1, 2015	1 Lakh crore	Digitally Empowered Nation	Aims to ensure that government services are available to citizens electronically and people get benefited from the latest information and communication technology
Gramin Bhandaran Yojna	MoA	March 31, 2007		Agriculture	Creation of scientific storage capacity with allied facilities in rural areas to meet the requirements of farmers for storing farm produce, processed farm produce and agricultural inputs. Improve their marketability through promotion of grading, standardization and quality control of agricultural produce
Indra Awaas Yojana	MoRD	1985		Housing, Rural	Provides financial assistance to rural poor for constructing their houses themselves
Indira Gandhi Matritva Sahyog Yojana	MoWCD	2010		Mother Care	A cash incentive of ₹4000 to women (19 years and above) for the first two live births

Contd...

Scheme	Ministry	Date of launch	Outlay/ Status	Sector	Provisions
Integrated Child Development Services	MoWCD	October 2, 1975		Child Development	Tackle malnutrition and health problems in children below 6 years of age and their mothers
Integrated Rural Development Program	MoRD	1978		Rural Development	Self-employment program to raise the income-generation capacity of target groups among the poor and the scheme has been merged with another scheme named Swarnajayanti Gram Swarozgar Yojana (SGSY) since 01/04/1999
Janani Suraksha Yojana	MoHFW	2005		Mother Care	One-time cash incentive to pregnant women for institutional/home births through skilled assistance
Jawaharlal Nehru National Urban Renewal Mission (JnNURM)	MoUD	December 3, 2005		Urban Development	To improve the quality of life and infrastructure in the cities. To be replaced by Atal Mission for Rejuvenation and Urban Transformation
Kasturba Gandhi Balika Vidyalaya	MoHRD	July 2004		Education	Educational facilities (residential schools) for girls belonging to SC, ST, OBC, minority communities and families below the poverty line (BPL) in Educationally Backward Blocks
INSPIRE Program	Department of Science and Technology (India)				Scholarships for top science students, fellowships for pursuing PhD, research grants to researchers
Kishore Vaigyanik Protsahan Yojana	MoST	1999			Scholarship program to encourage students to take up research careers in the areas of basic sciences, engineering and medicine
Livestock Insurance Scheme (India)	MoA			Education	Insurance to cattle and attaining qualitative improvement in livestock and their products
Mahatma Gandhi National Rural Employment Guarantee Act	MoRD	February 6, 2006	₹40,000 crore in 2010–11	Rural Wage Employment	Legal guarantee for one hundred days of employment in every financial year to adult members of any rural household willing to do public work-related unskilled manual work at the statutory minimum wage of ₹120 per day in 2009 prices

Contd...

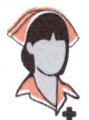

Scheme	Ministry	Date of launch	Outlay/ Status	Sector	Provisions
Members of Parliament Local Area Development Scheme	MoSPI	December 23, 1993			Each MP has the choice to suggest to the District Collector for, works to the tune of ₹5 crore per annum to be taken up in his/her constituency. The Rajya Sabah Member of Parliament can recommend works in one or more districts in the State from where he/she has been elected
Mid-day Meal Scheme	MoHRD	August 15, 1995		Health, Education	Lunch (free of cost) to school-children on all working days
Namami Gange Program	MoWR	March 1995	20,000 crore for 5 years	Clean and Protect Ganga	Integrates the efforts to clean and protect the river Ganga in a comprehensive manner
National Literacy Mission Program	MoHRD	May 5, 1988		Education	Make 80 million adults in the age group of 15–35 literate
National Pension Scheme		January 1, 2004		Pension	Contribution based pension system
National Scheme on Welfare of Fishermen	MoA			Agriculture	Financial assistance to fishers for construction of house, community hall for recreation and common working place and installation of tube wells for drinking water
National Service Scheme	MoYAS		1969		Personality development through social (or community) service
National Social Assistance Scheme	MoRD	August 15, 1995		Pension	Public assistance to its citizens in case of unemployment, old age, sickness and disablement and in other cases of undeserved want
Pooled Finance Development Fund Scheme	MOUD		2006	Agriculture and villagers welfare	Facilitate development of bankable urban and rural infrastructure projects financial help to urban local Bodies.
Pradhan Mantri Adarsh Gram Yojana	MoRD	July 23, 2010		Model Village	Integrated development of schedule caste majority villages in four states
Pradhan Mantri Suraksha Bima Yojana	MoF	May 9, 2015		Insurance	Accidental Insurance with a premium of ₹12 per year
Pradhan Mantri Jeevan Jyoti Bima Yojana	MoF	May 9, 2015		Insurance	Life insurance of ₹2 lakh with a premium of ₹330 per year

Contd...

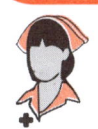

Scheme	Ministry	Date of launch	Outlay/ Status	Sector	Provisions
Pradhan Mantri Jan Dhan Yojana	MoF	August 28, 2014		Financial Inclusion	National mission for financial inclusion to ensure access to financial services, namely banking savings and deposit accounts remittance, credit, insurance, pension in an affordable manner
Pradhan Mantri Gram Sadak Yojana	MoRD	December 25, 2000		Rural Development	Good all-weather road connectivity to unconnected villages
Rajiv Awas Yojana	MhUPA	2013		Urban Housing	It envisages a "Slum Free India" with inclusive and equitable cities in which every citizen has access to basic civic infrastructure and social amenities and decent shelter
Rajiv Gandhi Grameen Vidyutikaran Yojana	MoP	April 2005	To be replaced by Deen Dayal Upadhyaya Gram Jyoti Yojana	Rural Electrification	Program for creation of Rural Electricity Infrastructure and Household Electrification for providing access to electricity to rural households
Rashtriya Krishi Vikas Yojana	MoA	August 1, 2007		Agricultural	Achieve 4% annual growth in agriculture through development of agriculture and its allied sectors during the XI plan period
Rashtriya Swasthya Bima Yojana	MoHFW	April 1, 2008		Insurance	Health insurance to poor (BPL), Domestic workers, MGNREGA workers, Rikshawpullers, building and other construction workers, and many other categories as may be identified by the respective states
RNTCP	MoHFW	1997		Health	Tuberculosis control initiative
Saksham or Rajiv Gandhi Scheme for Empowerment of Adolescent Boys	MoWCD	2014		Skill Development	Aims at all-round development of adolescent boys and make them self-reliant, gender sensitive and aware citizens, when they grow up. It covers all adolescent boys (both schools going and out of school) in the age group of 11 to 18 years subdivided into two categories, viz. 11–14 and 14–18 years. In 2014–15, an allocation of ₹25 crore is made for the scheme

Contd...

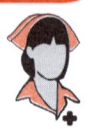

Scheme	Ministry	Date of launch	Outlay/ Status	Sector	Provisions
Sabla or Rajiv Gandhi Scheme for Empowerment of Adolescent Girls	MoWCD	2011		Skill Development	Empowering adolescent girls (age) of 11–18 years with focus on out-of-school girls by improvement in their nutritional and health status and upgrading various skill like home skills, life skills and vocational skills. Merged Nutrition Program for Adolescent Girls (NPAG) and Kishori Shakti Yojana (KSY)
Sampoorna Grameen Rozgar Yojana	MoRD	September 25, 2001		Rural Self-employment	Providing additional wage employment and food security, alongside creation of durable community assets in rural areas
Swabhiman	MoF	February 15, 2011		Financial Inclusion	To make banking facility available to all citizens and to get 5 crore accounts opened by March 2012, Replaced by Pradhan Mantri Jan Dhan Yojana
Swarnajayanti Gram Swarozgar Yojana	MoRD	April 1, 1999		Rural Employment	Bring the assisted poor families above the poverty line by organizing them into Self-Help Groups (SHGs) through the process of social mobilization, their training and capacity building and provision of income generating assets through a mix of bank credit and government subsidy
Swavalamban	MoF	September 26, 2010	To be replaced by Atal Pension Yojana	Pension	Pension scheme to the workers in unorganized sector. Any citizen who is not part of any statutory pension scheme of the government and contributes between ₹1000 and ₹12000/- per annum, could join the scheme. The Central Government shall contribute ₹1000 per annum to such subscribers
Udisha	MoWCD			Child Care	Training program for ICDS workers
Voluntary Disclosure of Income Scheme		June 18, 1997	Closed on December 31, 1998		Opportunity to the income tax/ wealth tax defaulters to disclose their undisclosed income at the prevailing tax rates
National Rural Livelihood Mission (NRLM)	MoRD	June 2011	$5.1 Billion		This scheme will organize rural poor into Self-Help Group (SHG) groups and make them capable for self-employment. The idea is to develop better livelihood options for the poor

Contd...

Scheme	Ministry	Date of launch	Outlay/ Status	Sector	Provisions
HRIDAY-Heritage City Development and Augmentation Yojana	MoUD	January 2015		Urban Development	The scheme seeks to preserve and rejuvenate the rich cultural heritage of the country
Sukanya Samridhi Yojana (Girl Child Prosperity Scheme)	MoWCD	January 2015			The scheme primarily ensures equitable share to a girl child in resources and savings of a family in which she is generally discriminated as against a male child
Smart Cities Mission	MoUD	June 25, 2015		Urban Development	To enable better living and drive economic growth stressing on the need for people centric urban planning and development
Atal Mission for Rejuvenation and Urban Transformation (AMRUT)	MoUD	June 25, 2015		Urban Development	To enable better living and drive economic growth stressing on the need for people centric urban planning and development
Pradhan Mantri Awas Yojana (PMAY)	MoUD	June 25, 2015		Housing	To enable better living and drive economic growth stressing on the need for people centric urban planning and development
National Child Labor Projects (NCLP)	Ministry of Labor and Employment	Lunched in 9 districts in 1987 and has been expanded in January 2005 to 250 districts in 21 different states of the country			The objective of this project is to eliminate child labor in hazardous industries by 2010. Under this scheme, the target group is all children below 14 years of age who are working in occupations and processes listed in the Schedule to the Child Labor (Prohibition and Regulation) Act, 1986 or occupations and processes that are harmful to the health of the child

Contd...

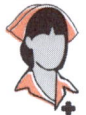

Scheme	Ministry	Date of launch	Outlay/ Status	Sector	Provisions
Antyodaya Anna Yojna	NDA Government	December 25, 2000			Under the scheme 1 crore of the poorest among the (Below Poverty Line) BPL families covered under the targeted public distribution system are identified. Issue of Ration Cards following the recognition of Antyodaya families, unique quota cards to be recognized an "Antyodaya Ration Card" must be given to the Antyodaya families by the chosen power. The scheme has been further expanded twice by additional 50 lakh BPL families each in June 2003 and in August 2004, thus covering 2 crore families under the AAY scheme
National Food Security Mission	Government of India	2007 for 5 years			It launched in 2007 for 5 years to increase production and productivity of wheat, rice and pulses on a sustainable basis so as to ensure food security of the country. The aim is to bridge the yield gap in respect of these crops through dissemination of improved technologies and farm management practices.

EMPLOYEES STATE INSURANCE (ESI)

The ESI Act passed in 1948 (ESI act amended in 1975, 1984, 1989, 2006 and 2017) is an important measure of social security and health insurance in this country. It provides for certain cash and medical benefits to industrial employees in case of sickness, maternity and employment injury.

Scope

The Act extends to the whole of India. The ESI Act of 1948 covered all power using factories other than reasonable factories wherein 200 or more persons were employed (excluding mines, railways, and defence establishments). The provisions of the ESI (Amendment) Act of 1975 were extended to the following new classes of establishments:

- Small power using factories employing 10–19 persons and non-power using factories employing 20 or more persons.
- Shops.
- Hotel and restaurants.
- Cinemas and theaters.
- Road motor transport establishments
- Newspaper establishments.

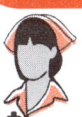

With effect from 1.10.2006 the Act covers all employee's manual, clerical, supervisory and technical getting up to ₹10,000 per month. The provisions of the Act can be extended to any other agricultural or commercial establishments.

Administration

The administration of the ESI scheme under the Act is entrusted to an autonomous body called the ESI Corporation. The Union Minister for Labor is the Chairman and the Secretary of Government of India, Ministry of Labor is the Vice Chairman of this Corporation. It consists of members representing central and state governments, employers and employees organizations, medical profession and Parliament. There is a standing committee, constituted from the members of the Corporation, which act as an executive body for the administration of the scheme. The chief executive officer of the corporation is the Director General who is assisted by four principal officers.

1. Insurance commissioner.
2. Medical commissioner.
3. Financial commissioner.
4. **Statutory Body:** There is a Medical Benefit Council which is headed by the Director General of health services. Government of India who is assisted by the Medical Commissioner in all matters relating to medical relief.

Finance

This scheme is run by contributions of employees and employers and grants from central and state governments.

The employer contributes 4.75% of total wage bill; the employee contributes 1.75% of wages.

Benefits to Employees

The Act has made provision for the following benefits to insured persons or to other dependants as the case may be:

- Medical benefit
- Sickness benefit
- Maternity benefit
- Disablement benefit
- Dependent's benefit
- Funeral expenses
- Rehabilitation allowance

Benefits to Employers

- Exemption from the applicability of Workmen's Compensation Act, 1923.
- Exemption from Maternity Benefit Act, 1961.
- Exemption from payment of medical allowance to employees and their dependents or arranging for their medical care.
- Rebate under the Income Tax Act on contribution deposited in the ESI account.
- Healthy workforce.

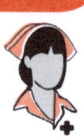

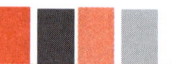

ASSESS YOURSELF

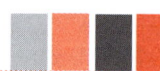

1. Write the types of cost.
2. Explain about ESI.
3. What are five-year plans? What are your responsibilities as nurse for five-year plans?
4. Explain minimum need program.

Index

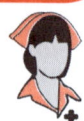

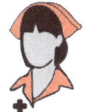

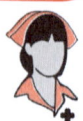